Special Issue
Included in subscription

Pediatric Neurosurgery (ISSN 1016–2291), **Vol. 18, No. 2 (1992)**
Editor: F.J. Epstein, New York, N.Y.

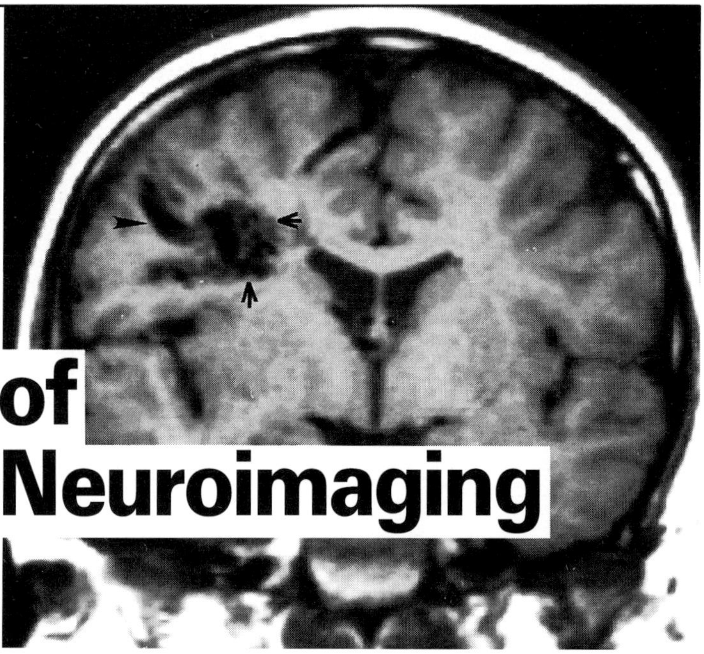

Horizons of Pediatric Neuroimaging

Editor:
Robert A. Zimmerman, Philadelphia, Pa.

The vast improvements in neuroimaging techniques made during the 1980's have brought tremendous benefits to neurosurgery. In this special issue, leading neurosurgeons review the various applications of new neuroimaging techniques in pediatric neurology. The contributions of magnetic resonance to the diagnosis of intracranial infection and of pediatric posterior fossa tumors as well as the intraoperative uses of ultrasound in the pediatric patient are reviewed. In addition, current perspectives on the evaluation of hydrocephalus and on the utility of different imaging modalities in epileptic surgical candidates are presented.

Contents

Fields of Interest
Neurosurgery, Neuroscience, Radiology

Horizons of Pediatric Neuroimaging
'Pediatric Neurosurgery', Vol. 18, No. 2 (1992)
Editor: Zimmerman, R.A. (Philadelphia, Pa.)
64 p., 66 fig., 2 cpl., 4 tab., soft cover, 1992
SFr. 55.– / DM 66.– / £ 27.50 / US $ 44.00
Prices subject to change
DM price for FRG, £ price for UK, US $ price for USA only
ISBN 3-8055-5694-2

KI 92172

KARGER

Stereotactic and Functional Neurosurgery

Official Journal of the World Society for Stereotactic and Functional Neurosurgery

Official Journal of the American Society for Stereotactic and Functional Neurosurgery

Founded 1938 as 'Confinia Neurologica' by E.A. Spiegel
Continued 1975–1988 as 'Applied Neurophysiology'

Publication data: 'Stereotactic and Functional Neurosurgery' is published 8 times annually. Volumes 60–61 with 4 issues each appear in 1993.

Subscription rates: Subscriptions run for a full calendar year. Prices are given per volume.

Personal subscription:
Subscription + postage and handling
SFr. 151.20 + SFr. 11.20 Europe
SFr. 151.20 + SFr. 16.80 Overseas
US$ 100.80 + US$ 11.20
(Must be in the name of, billed to, and paid by an individual. Order must be marked 'personal subscription'.)

Institutional subscription:
Subscription + postage and handling
SFr. 216.– + SFr. 16.– Europe
SFr. 216.– + SFr. 24.– Overseas
US$ 144.00 + US$ 16.00

Airmail postage: SFr. 24.–, US$ 20.00. (Extra per volume.)

Discount subscription prices: Societies for Stereotactic and Functional Neurosurgery are requested to apply for appropriate discounts.

Microform edition: SFr. 108.–, US$ 72.00. (Available exclusively to subscribers of the paper edition.)

Subscription orders: Orders can be placed at agencies, bookstores, directly with the Publisher S. Karger AG, P.O. Box, CH-4009 Basel (Switzerland) or with any of the following distributors:

Deutschland: S. Karger GmbH
Lörracher Strasse 16A, Postfach
D-W-7800 Freiburg

France: Librairie Luginbühl
36, bd de Latour-Maubourg
F-75007 Paris

Great Britain, Ireland: S. Karger Publishers
11 Ravenscroft Road
Beckenham, Kent BR3 4TP

USA: S. Karger Publishers, Inc.
26 West Avon Road, P.O. Box 529
Farmington, CT 06085

India, Bangladesh, Sri Lanka:
S. Karger India Subscription Agency
B-5/132 Safdarjung Enclave
New Delhi-110029

Japan: Katakura Libri, Inc.
36-9 Hongo 3-chome, Bunkyo-ku
Tokyo 113

Change of address: Both old and new address should be sent to the subscription source.

Single issues and back volumes: Information can be obtained through the Publisher.

Bibliographic indices: This journal is regularly listed in bibliographic services, including *Current Contents®*.

Book Reviews: Books are accepted for review by special agreement.

Advertising: Correspondence and rate requests should be addressed to the Publisher.

KARGER

Stereotact Funct Neurosurg
Printed in Switzerland by
Basler Zeitung AG, Basel

S. Karger AG,
Postfach, CH-4009 Basel (Schweiz)

Erscheint anderthalbmonatlich;
pro Jahr 2 Bände zu 4 Heften

Stereotactic and Functional Neurosurgery

Submission: Only original papers written in English are considered and should be sent to:

Prof. Dr. Ph.L. Gildenberg
6560 Fannin Street, Suite 1530
Houston, TX 77030 (USA)

Manuscripts should be submitted in triplicate (with three sets of illustrations of which one is an original), typewritten double-spaced on one side of the paper, with a wide margin.

Conditions: All manuscripts are subjected to editorial review. Manuscripts are received with the explicit understanding that they are not under simultaneous consideration by any other publication. Submission of an article for publication implies the transfer of the copyright from the author to the publisher upon acceptance. Accepted papers become the permanent property of 'Stereotactic and Functional Neurosurgery' and may not be reproduced by any means, in whole or in part, without the written consent of the publisher. It is the author's responsibility to obtain permission to reproduce illustrations, tables, etc. from other publications.

Arrangement:

Title page: The first page of each paper should indicate the title (main title underlined), the authors' names, and the institute where the work was conducted. A short title for use as running head as well as the full address of the author to whom correspondence should be sent are also required.

Full address: The exact postal address complete with postal code of the senior author must be given at the bottom of the title page. Please also supply phone and fax numbers.

Key words: For indexing purposes, a list of 3–10 key words in English is essential.

Abstract: Each paper needs an abstract of up to 10 lines.

Small type: Paragraphs which can or must be set in smaller type (case histories, test methods, etc.) should be indicated with a 'p' (petit) in the margin on the left-hand side.

Footnotes: Avoid footnotes. When essential, they are numbered consecutively and typed at the foot of the appropriate page.

Tables and illustrations: Tables and illustrations (both numbered in Arabic numerals) should be prepared on separate sheets. Tables require a heading and figures a legend, also prepared on a separate sheet. For the reproduction of illustrations, only good drawings and original photographs can be accepted; negatives or photocopies cannot be used. When possible, group several illustrations on one block for reproduction (max. size 113 × 174 mm) or provide crop marks. On the back of each illustration, indicate its number, the author's name, and 'top'. Color illustrations are reproduced at the author's expense.

References: In the text identify references by Arabic numerals [in square brackets]. Material submitted for publication but not yet accepted should be noted as 'unpublished data' and not be included in the reference list. The list of references should include only those publications which are cited in the text. Do not alphabetize; number references in the order in which they are first mentioned in the text. The surnames of the authors followed by initials should be given. There should be no punctuation other than a comma to separate the authors. Cite all authors, 'et al' is not sufficient. Abbreviate journal names according to the Index Medicus system. (Also see International Committee of Medical Journal Editors: Uniform requirements for manuscripts submitted to biomedical journals. Br Med J 1988;296: 401–405.)

Examples

(a) Papers published in periodicals: Kauffman HF, van der Heide S, Beaumont F, Blok H, de Vries K: Class-specific antibody determination against *Aspergillus fumigatus* by means of the enzyme-linked immunosorbent assay. III. Comparative study: IgG, IgA, IgM ELISA titers, precipitating antibodies and IgE binding after fractionation of the antigen. Int Arch Allergy Appl Immunol 1986;80:300–306.

(b) Monographs: Matthews DE, Farewell VT: Using and Understanding Medical Statistics. Basel, Karger, 1985.

(c) Edited books: Hardy WD Jr, Essex M: FeLV-induced feline acquired immune deficiency syndrome: A model for human AIDS; in Klein E (ed): Acquired Immunodeficiency Syndrome. Prog Allergy. Basel, Karger, 1986, vol 37, pp 353–376.

Further details: Authors may consult our leaflet 'Rules for the Preparation of Manuscripts', available on request from the Publisher, S. Karger AG, P.O. Box, CH-4009 Basel (Switzerland).

Page charges: There is no page charge for papers of 8 or fewer printed pages (including tables, illustrations and references). Each additional complete or partial page is charged to the author at SFr. 225.– / US $ 150.00. The allotted size of a paper is equal to approx. 16 manuscript pages (including tables, illustrations and references).

Galley proofs: Unless indicated otherwise, galley proofs are sent to the first-named author and should be returned with the least possible delay. Alterations made in galley proofs, other than the correction of printer's errors, are charged to the author. No page proofs are supplied.

Reprints: Order forms and a price list are sent with the galley proofs. Orders submitted after the issue is printed are subject to considerably higher prices. Allow five weeks from date of publication for delivery of reprints.

KARGER

Proceedings of the 2nd International Workshop on
Microphysiological Recordings during Stereotactic Neurosurgery

Motor Thalamus

October 1–2, 1989, Nikko, Japan

Editors
Chihiro Ohye, Maebayashi
Yoshikazu Shinoda, Tokyo
Philip L. Gildenberg, Houston, Tex.
Patricia O. Franklin, Houston, Tex.

51 figures, 1 table, 1993

KARGER

S. Karger · Medical and ientific Publishers
Basel · Freiburg · Paris · London · New York · New Delhi · Bangkok · Singapore · Tokyo · Sydney

---

Drug Dosage

The authors and the publisher have exerted every effort to ensure that drug selection and dosage set forth in this text are in accord with current recommendations and practice at the time of publication. However, in view of ongoing research, changes in government regulations, and the constant flow of information relating to drug therapy and drug reactions, the reader is urged to check the package insert for each drug for any change in indications and dosage and for added warnings and precautions. This is particularly important when the recommended agent is a new and/or infrequently employed drug.

Printed in Switzerland on acid-free paper by Basler Zeitung, Basel
ISBN 3-8055-5756-6

Contents

Proceedings of the 2nd International Workshop on Microphysiological Recordings during Stereotactic Neurosurgery: Motor Thalamus, October 1–2, 1989, Nikko, Japan
Stereotact Funct Neurosurg 1993;60:5

Preface

This special issue of *Stereotactic and Functional Neurosurgery* represents papers presented at the Second Meeting of the Stereotactic Microrecording Study Group held at Nikko, October 1–2, 1989, in combination with the 10th Meeting of the World Society for Stereotactic and Functional Neurosurgery in Maebashi, October 3–5, 1989. As the first meeting was held in Evian, France, in honor of Madame D. Albe-Fessard, mother of microrecording in the human thalamus, at the beautiful lakeside, we chose the second meeting site also here in a national park, Syuzenji Lake. Unfortunately, Madame Albe-Fessard was absent because of her illness. All the papers presented here under the main theme of 'Motor thalamus' were excellent, and many fruitful discussions were had during one and a half days of sessions.

The target area of our stereotactic intervention has long been, more or less, the ventrolateral thalamic zone. However, anatomical and functional classification of that area in the human thalamus is still debated. The widely used Hassler's classification, ventroanterior, ventro-oral anterior, ventro-oral posterior, ventrointermediate, ventrocaudal, in this order from rostral to caudal, is not always compatible with the classification in nonhuman primates, i.e., ventral anterior, ventral lateral oral, ventral lateral caudal, ventral posterior lateral and medial, also in order. Probably, one of the most difficult discrepancies is to define the equivalent of 'VL', the well-known motor thalamus in animals, in the human thalamus.

New facts and hypotheses were presented and discussed. Certainly, it was too early to draw a definite conclusion. Many problems still remain to be solved. There are agreements and disagreements, but we are sure that all the participants felt that we had made one step of progress toward better understanding of the human thalamus.

Chihiro Ohye

Proceedings of the 2nd International Workshop on Microphysiological Recordings during Stereotactic Neurosurgery: Motor Thalamus, October 1–2, 1989, Nikko, Japan
Stereotact Funct Neurosurg 1993;60:6–16

Comparative Anatomical Study of Ventrolateral Thalamic Mass in Humans and Monkeys

Tatsuo Hirai[a], *Edward G. Jones*[b]

[a] Department of Neurosurgery, Heisei Memorial Hospital, Shizuoka, Japan;
[b] Department of Anatomy and Neurobiology, University of California, Irvine, Calif., USA

Key Words. Human thalamus · Monkey thalamus · Cytometory · Acetylcholinesterase · Thalamus

Abstract. Cytoarchitecture and enzyme activity in the ventrolateral thalamic mass of humans and monkeys were examined using conventional Nissl, myelin stain and histochemical methods. According to the data obtained from cytometric analysis, the histogram patterns of cell dimensions and cell density in each ventrolateral thalamic nucleus in humans and monkeys were very similar. Moreover, acetylcholinesterase-stained sections revealed a parcellation of the ventrolateral thalamic nuclei that could be correlated with that in the monkey thalamus. Apart from differences of size, the nuclei of the human and monkey thalamus are remarkably similar. We proposed accordingly that a new parcellation of human thalamic nuclei be based on cytometric analysis and histochemical staining.

Introduction

Microelectrode recordings from human thalamic ventrolateral nuclei [1–3], made in the course of stereotactic thalamotomy for the treatment of involuntary movement disorders, including Parkinson's disease, make it possible to understand the functional properties of the human thalamic ventrolateral nuclei when compared with the functional properties of those of monkeys [4–6]. In order to ascertain physiological data which were very similar in both species, we conducted a comparative anatomical study of ventrolateral thalamic nuclei in both humans [7–10] and monkeys [4, 11, 12].

1011–6125/93/0603–0006 $ 2.75/0

Materials and Methods

Three human thalami from neurologically normal persons and three monkey thalami (Macaque) were fixed in 10% neutral formalin for at least 3 months for cytometric analysis. A square block containing the thalamus was cut from the brain and serial frozen sections were cut at 50 μm in the coronal, sagittal, or horizontal plane, referring to the intercommissural plane. The thalamic nuclei of the ventrolateral group were delineated, based on the dimensions and density of neurons in each group, by referring to Hassler's classification and terminology (fig. 1). Using a microscopic image analyzer (Olympus VIP-21CH), the number and dimensions of the neurons in selected protions (measuring 1 mm of each nucleus in humans and 0.5 mm in monkeys) were measured directly from the sections at 1,000 times magnification. A histogram was prepared for each nucleus.

Three human thalami from neurologically normal persons and three monkey thalami (Macaque) were fixed by 4% phosphate-buffered paraformaldehyde, sectioned, and frozen in frontal, sagittal or horizontal planes for histochemical study. Four of every five sections were cut at 30 μm and one of each was stained with acetylcholinesterase (AChE), cytochrome oxidase (CO), thionine and myeline. Sections from the thick thionine, AChE, CO and myelin series were examined under magnification over a range of 7.5–30, under a Wild dissecting microscope equipped with a camera lucida. Densities of histochemical staining were drawn using criteria previously agreed upon. Drawings of each trio of sections from the 3 series were superimposed, using blood vessel profiles as guides, the nuclear border was then traced on the drawing of the thionine-stained series.

Results

The Vim (nucleus ventrointermedius) nucleus of Hassler in humans is easily identified in horizontal and sagittal sections. It is distinguished from the other ventrolateral thalamic subnuclei as a relatively cell-sparse zone, which contains darkly stained large and medium-sized angular cells with areas of about 500–1,000 and 300–400 μm, respectively. The histogram shows two peaks of cell area around 600–700 and 400 μm and cell density in the nucleus is about 50–90/mm/50 μm. The AChE is negative in the Vim nucleus (fig. 2).

The VPLo (nucleus ventralis posterior lateralis pars oralis) nucleus of Olszewski in monkeys is easily identified in horizontal and sagittal sections as a cell-sparse zone. The VPLo nucleus contains darkly stained large and medium-sized cells with areas of about 400–800 and 200–400 μm, respectively. The cell density is about 40–60/0.25 mm/50 μm thickness. The AChE is negative in the VPLo nucleus.

The large cells, their sparse distribution, the position and shape of the Vim and VPLo nucleus and the negative AChE gives a remarkable

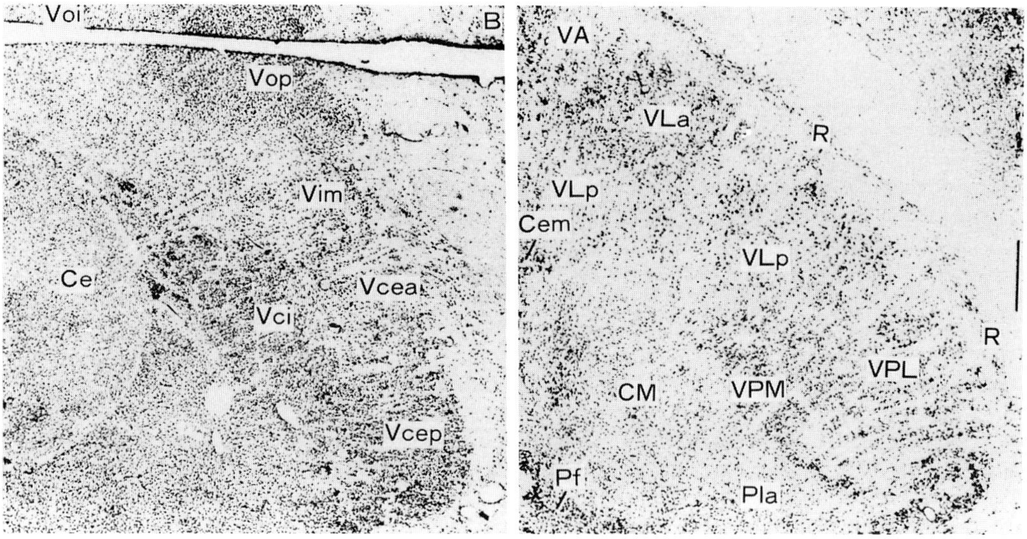

Fig. 1. Horizontal section through the ventrolateral thalamic nuclei of humans (left) and monkeys (right) showing the cytoarchitecture of each ventolateral thalamic nucleus under low-power magnification. Each ventrolateral thalamic nucleus is represented by Hassler's (humans) and Jones' (monkey) thalamic classification and terminology. Note that the cytoarchitecture of the human ventrolateral thalamic nuclei is very similar to that of the monkey.

similarity between Vim and VPLo nucleus [the greater part of the ventral lateral posterior nucleus (VLp) of Jones in the monkey].

The Voi (nucleus ventrooralis internus) of Hassler in humans is composed of large and medium neurons whose dimensions are about 400–600 and 300–400 μm, respectively. The histogram shows one peak around 400 μm. The cell density is about 70–100/mm/50 μm thickness and the AChE is negative in the Voi nucleus.

The nucleus X of Olszewski in monkeys consists mainly of loosely and evenly arranged large and medium neurons with areas about 300–600 and 200–300 μm, respectively. The cell density is about 70–80/0.25 μm/50 μm thickness and the AChE is negative in the Voi nucleus. The Voi nucleus appears to correspond to nucleus X of Olszewski and to the internal part of the ventral lateral posterior nucleus (VLp) of Jones.

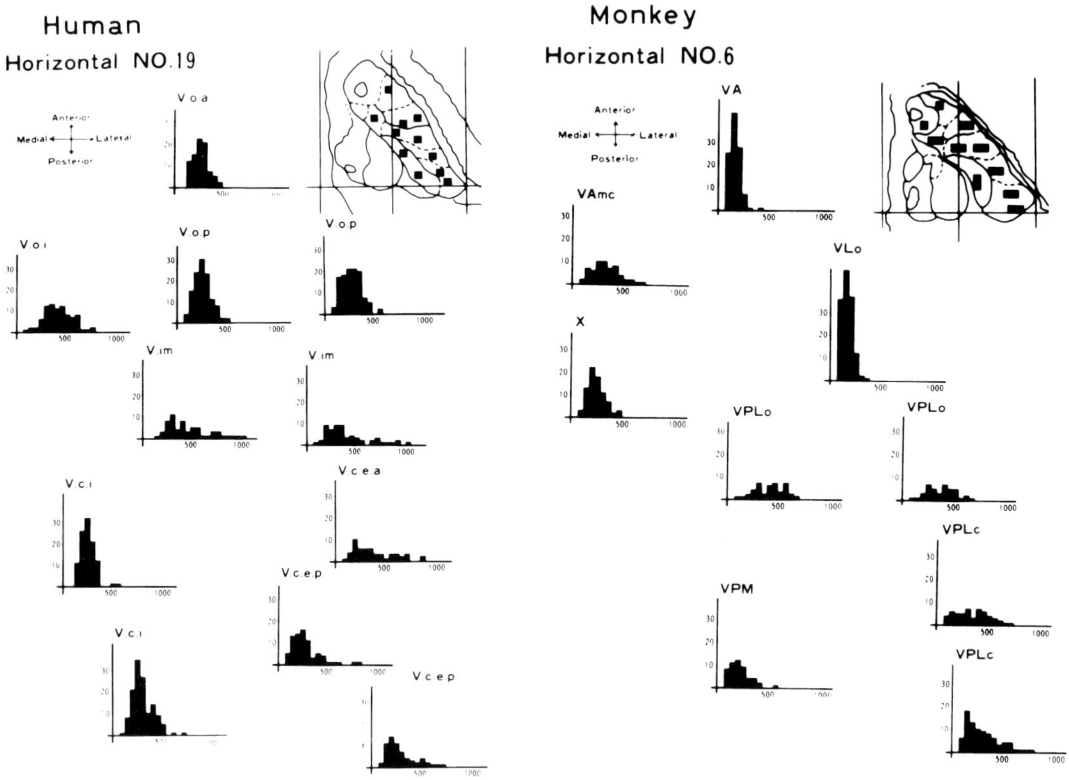

Fig. 2. The histogram of cell dimension and density in a 1-mm area (humans) and a 0.25-mm area (monkeys) in various ventrolateral thalamic nuclei about 1.9 mm (humans) and 0.6 mm (monkeys) above the intercommissure line in the horizontal section. In each of the right upper drawings of the thalamus, the horizontal line is drawn at the level of the posterior commissure and the three vertical lines indicate the midline, 10 mm, 20 mm (humans) or midline, 5 mm, 10 mm (monkeys) from the midline. The histograms are distributed in a manner corresponding to the positions of the black squares on each of the upper right drawings. In each histogram, the abscissa represents the cell deminsion (μm) and the ordinate represents the number of cells per 1 mm (humans) and 0.25 mm (monkeys). Note in both species that the cell-sparse zone is rich in large neurons but less densely arranged. Each thalamic nucleus is represented by Hassler's (humans) and Olszewski's (monkeys) terminology.

Together, the Vim, Voi, Zim (nucleus zentrointermedius) and Dim (nucleus dorsointermedius) nuclei probably correspond to the nucleus VPLo, nucleus X, VLc (nucleus ventrolateralis pars caudalis) and VLpc (nucleus ventralis pars parvocelluralis) of Olszewski or to the ventral lateral posterior nucleus (VLp) of Jones.

The Voa (nucleus ventro-oralis anterior) and Vop (nucleus ventro-oralis posterior) nucleis of Hassler in humans consist mainly of densely packed moderately stained medium and medium-small neurons about 300–400 and 200–300 μm in area, respectively. The histogram of these shows one paek around 250 μm. The cell density is about 80–160/mm/50 μm thickness in the Voa nucleus and about 80–150/mm/50 μm thickness in the Vop nucleus. These nuclei give the appearance of considerable uniformity and the AChE is strongly positive in both the Voa and the Vop nucleus (fig. 3a).

The VLo (nuclus ventralis lateralis pars oralis) nucleus of Olszewski in monkeys consists mainly of densely packed clustered medium and medium-small neurons with areas of about 150–450 and 100–250 μm, respectively. The cell density is about 90–150/0.25 mm/50 μm thickness and the AChE is strongly positive in the VLo nucleus (fig. 3b).

Together, the Voa, Vop, Zo (nucleus zentrooralis) and Do (nucleus dorzooralis) nuclei probably correspond to the nucleus ventralis lateralis pars oralis (VLo) of Olszewski or to the ventral lateral anterior nucleus (VLa) of Jones.

The Vci (nucleus ventrocaudalis internus) nucleus of Hassler in humans is composed of small, medium-small and medium-sized neurons compactly arranged in clumps with areas varying between 100 and 500 μm. The histogram shows one peak around 300 μm. The cell density is about 90–150/mm/50 μm thickness. AChE is moderately positive.

The VPM (nucleus ventralis posterior medialis) nucleus of Olszewski in monkeys is composed of small, medium-small and medium-sized neurons arranged in clusters, with areas varying from 100 to 500 μm. The cell density is about 90–120/0.25 mm/50 μm thickness. The AChE is moderately positive in the VPM nucleus.

The Vce (nucleus ventrocaudalis externus) of Hassler in humans contains neurons which exhibit considerable morphological differences. There are small, medium-small, medium and large neurons, whose dimensions vary from 100 to 1,000 μm. The histogram shows two peaks around 200–300 and 450–550 μm. Two parts of the nucleus can be discerned, but there is no clear border between them. An anterior compo-

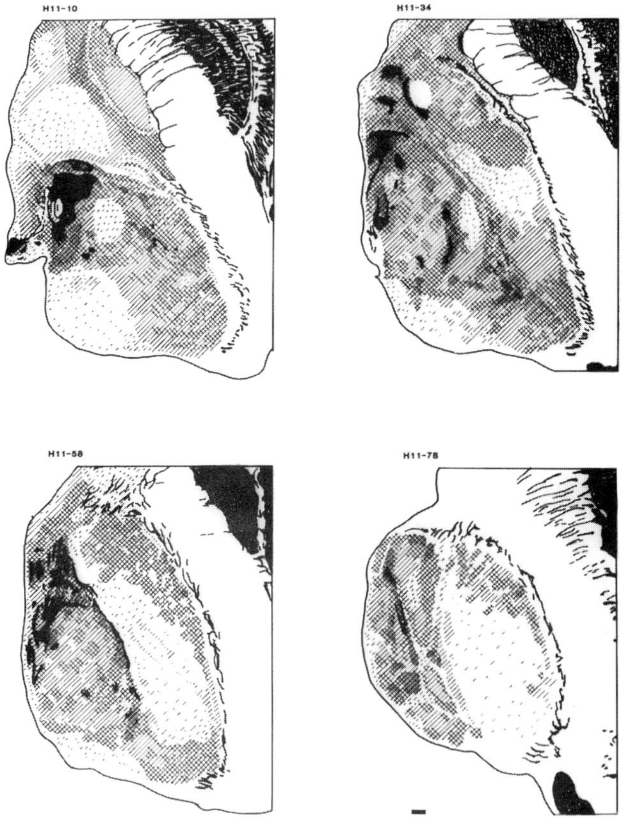

3a

Fig. 3. a Distribution patterns of AChE activity in human horizontal sections. The sections are arranged from ventral to dorsal. **b** Distribution patterns of AChE activity in monkey coronal sections. The sections are arranged from anterior to posterior. Note that the cell-sparse zone in both human and monkey thalamus is AChE negative.

nent (Vcea: nucleus ventrocaudalis externus anterior) contains less densely packed, large cells, while a posterior component (Vcep: nucleus ventrocaudalis externus posterior) contains the full range of cell sizes which are more densely packed. The cell density in the Vcea nucleus is about 50–100/mm/50 μm thickness and the Vcep nucleus is about 70–160/mm/50 μm thickness. The AChE is moderately positive in both the Vcea and the Vcep nucleus.

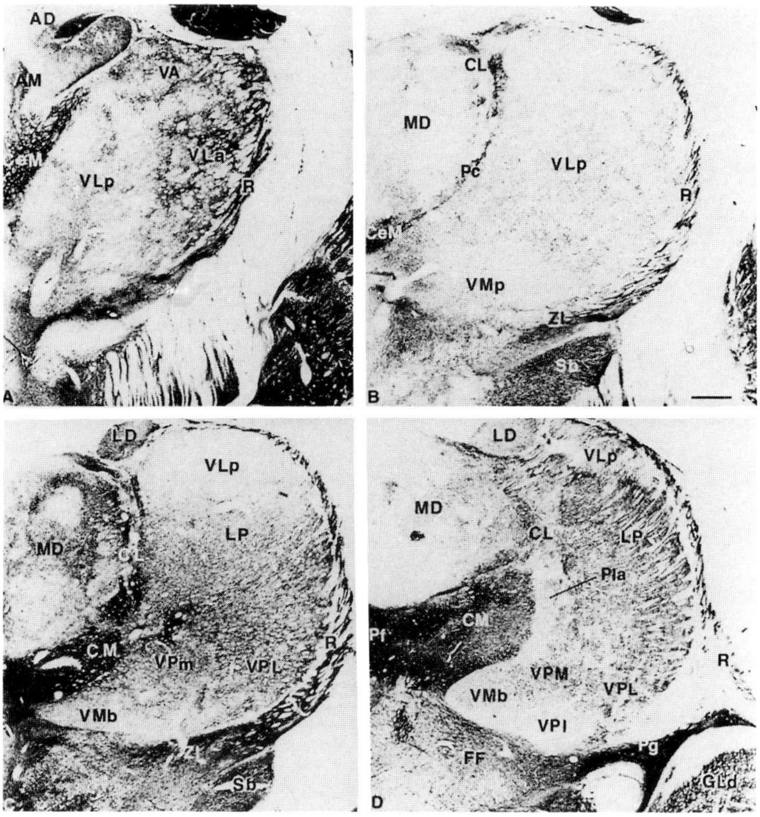

3b

The VPLc (nucleus ventralis posterior lateralis pars caudalis) nucleus of Olszewski in monkeys is composed of small, medium-small, medium and large neurons, whose areas are between 100 and 800 μm. The anterior part of the nucleus is loosely arranged and the cell density is about 55–85/0.25 mm/50 μm thickness. By contrast, the posterior part of the nucleus is more compactly arranged with medium and small neurons. The cell density is about 90–120/0.25 mm/50 μm thickness.

The Vci and Vce nuclei correspond, respectively, to the nucleus ventralis posterior medialis (VPM) and nucleus ventralis posterior lateralis pars caudalis (VPLc) of Olszewski and to the ventral posterior

Table 1. Correlation between the terminology of the ventrolateral thalamic nuclei in humans and monkeys

Jones' terminology			
AD	anterodorsal nucleus	Pla	anterior pulvinar nucleus
AM	anteromedial nucleus	R	reticular nucleus
CL	central lateral nucleus	VA	ventral anterior nucleus
CeM	central medial nucleus	VLa	ventral lateral anterior nucleus
CM	centre median nucleus	VLp	ventral lateral posterior nucleus
GLd	dorsal lateral geniculate nucleus	VM	ventral midial nucleus
LD	lateral dorsal nucleus	VMb	basal ventral medial nucleus
LP	lateral posterior nucleus	VPI	ventral posterior inferior nucleus
MD	mediodorsal nucleus	VPL	ventral posterior lateral nucleus
Pc	paracentral nucleus	VPM	ventral posterior medial nucleus
Pf	parafascicular nucleus	ZI	zona incerta
Hassler's terminology			
Lpo	nucleus lateropolaris thalami	Vci	nucleus ventrocaudalis internus
Dim	nucleus dorzointermedius	Voa	nucleus ventrooralis anterior
Do	nucleus dorzooralis	Voi	nucleus ventrooralis internus
Vim	nucleus ventrointermedius	Vop	nucleus ventrooralis posterior
Vcea	nucleu ventrocaudalis externus anterior	Zim	nucleus zentrointermedius
		Zo	nucleus zentrooralis
Vcep	nucleus ventrocaudalis externus posterior		
Olszewski's terminology			
VA	nucleus ventralis anterior	VPM	nucleus ventralis posterior medialis
VAmc	nucleus ventralis anterior magnocellularis	VPLc	nucleus ventralis posterior lateralis pars caudalis
VLc	nucleus ventralis lateralis pars caudalis	VPLo	nucleus ventralis posterior lateralis pars oralis
VLo	nucleus ventralis lateralis pars oralis	X	nucleus X
VLpc	nucleus ventralis lateralis pars parvocelluralis		

medial nucleus (VPM) and ventral posterior lateral nucleus (VPL) of Jones.

Correlation between the terminology of the ventrolateral thalamic nuclei in humans and monkeys is shown in table 1.

Discussion

According to the data obtained from cytometric analysis [13], the histogram patterns of cell dimensions and cell density in each ventrolateral thalamic nucleus in both humans and monkeys were very similar. Moreover, acetylcholinesterase-stained sections revealed a parcellation of the ventrolateral thalamic nuclei that could be correlated with that used in the monkey thalamus [14–16].

The Vim, Voi, Zim and Dim nuclei of Hassler [9] in humans compose a large cell-sparse zone comparative to VLp nucleus of Jones [4] in monkeys, which is equivalent to VPLo, nucleus X, VLc and VLpc nuclei of Olszewski in monkey. The AChE is negative in the cell-sparse zone of humans and monkeys. The Voa, Vop, Zo, and Do nuclei of Hassler in humans compose one nucleus comparative to the VLa nucleus of Jones in monkeys, which is equivalent to the VLo nucleus of Olszewski in monkeys, in which the AChE is strongly positive. The Vci, Vce nuclei of Hassler in humans comprise the specific sensory nucleus, comparable to the VPM and VPL nuclei of Jones in monkeys, which are equivalent to VPM and VPLc of Olszewski in monkeys, in which AChE is moderately positive.

The functional properties of the human thalamic ventrolateral nuclei should be taken into consideration to be compared with the functional properties of those of monkeys. It has now become clear from experimental studies in monkeys [4–6, 11] that VLa, VLp and VPL nuclei represent the respective thalamic relays for the globus pallidus, deep cerebellar nuclei and medial lemniscus, and that there is no overlap in the terminations of these 3 great afferent pathways. The VLa, VLp and VPL/VPM clearly project, without overlap, to different cortical areas, which may be loosely defined as premotor, motor and somatosensory, respectively, although the full details of the VLa projection are incompletely known.

Consequently, from these comparative anatomical studies, it is natural to consider that the deep sensory responses obtained by microelectrode recordings from the human thalamic ventrolateral nucleus might be localized in the VPLa nucleus (anterodorsal part of VPL nucleus), which is equivalent to the Vcea nucleus of Hassler, and the cutaneous sensory responses might be distributed in the VPLp nucleus (the core of the VPL nucleus), which is equivalent to the Vcep nucleus of Hassler. Moreover, the tremor-locked discharges [2, 3] in patients with movement disorders are perhaps more consistent with the predominant cerebellar input to the VLp nucleus, which is equivalent to the Vim nucleus of Hassler. Nissl and acetylcholinesterase-stained sections revealed a clear parcellation of the ventrolateral nuclei that could be correlated with that used in the Macaque monkey thalamus. Human nuclei were accordingly renamed using the monkey nomenclature of Jones [14, 15].

References

1 Lenz FA, Dostrovsky JO, Tasker RR, Yamashiro K, Kwan HC, Murphy JT: Single-unit analysis of the human ventral thalamic nuclear group: Somatosensory responses. J Neurophysiol 1988;59:299–316.
2 Lenz FA, Tasker RR, Kwan HC, Schnider S, Kwong R, Murayama Y, Dostrovsky JO, Murphy JT: Single unit analysis of the human ventral thalamic nuclear group: Correlation of thalamic tremor cells with the 3–6 Hz component of Parkinsonian tremor. J Neurosci 1988;8:754–764.
3 Ohye C, Shibazaki T, Hirai T, Wada H, Hirato M, Kawashima Y: Further physiological observations on the ventralis intermedius neurons in the human thalamus. J Neurophysiol 1989;61:488–500.
4 Jones EG: The Thalamus. New York, Plenum Press, 1985.
5 Jones EG, Friedman DP, Hendry SHC: Thalamic basis of place and modality-specific columns in monkey somatosensory cortex: A correlative anatomical and physiological study. J Neurophysiol 1982;48:545–568.
6 Jones EG, Wise SP, Coulter JD: Differential thalamic relationships of sensory motor and parietal cortical fields in monkeys. J Comp Neurol 1979;183:833–882.
7 Dewulf A: Anatomy of the Normal Human Thalamus, Topometry and Standardized Nomenclature. Amsterdem, Elsevier, 1971.
8 Emmers R, Tasker RR: The Human Somesthetic Thalamus, with Maps for Physiological Target Localization during Stereotaxic Neurosurgery. New York, Raven Press, 1970.
9 Hassler R: Anatomy of the Thalamus; in Schaltenbrand G, Bailey P (eds): Introduction to Stereotaxis with an Atlas of the Human Brain. Stuttgart, Thieme, 1959, pp 230–290.
10 Van Buren JM, Borke RC: Variations and Connections of the Human Thalamus. Berlin, Springer, 1972.

11 Ilinsky IA, Kultas-Ilinsky K: Sagittal cytoarchitectonic maps of the *Macaca mulatta* thalamus with a revised nomenclature of the motor-related nuclei validated by observations on their connectivity. J Comp Neurol 1987;262:331–364.

12 Olszewski J: The Thalamus of the *Macaca mulatta*. An Atlas for Use with the Stereotaxic Instrument. Basel, Karger, 1952.

13 Hirai T, Ohye C, Nagaseki Y, Matsumura M: Cytometric analysis of the thalamic ventralis intermedius nucleus in man and a comparison with the monkey. J Neurophysiol 1989;61:478–487.

14 Hirai T, Jones EG: A new parcellation of the human thalamus on the basis of histochemical staining. Brain Res Rev 1989;14:1–34.

15 Hirai T, Jones EG: Distribution of tachykinin and enkephalin immunoreactive fibers in the human thalamus. Brain Res Rev 1989;14:35–52.

16 Jones EG, Hendry SHC, Brandon C: Cytochrome oxidase staining reveals functional organization of monkey somatosensory thalamus. Exp Brain Res 1986;62: 438–442.

Dr. T. Hirai, Department of Neurosurgery, Heisei Memorial Hospital,
123-1 Mizukami, Fujieda, Shizuoka T426 (Japan)

Proceedings of the 2nd International Workshop on Microphysiological Recordings during Stereotactic Neurosurgery: Motor Thalamus, October 1–2, 1989, Nikko, Japan
Stereotact Funct Neurosurg 1993;60:17–31

Input-Output Organization of the Ventrolateral Nucleus of the Thalamus

Y. Shinoda, T. Futami, S. Kakei

Department of Physiology, School of Medicine, Tokyo Medical and Dental University, Yushima, Bunkyo-ku, Tokyo, Japan

Key Words. Thalamus · Ventrolateral nucleus · Motor cortex · Cerebellum

Abstract. Input-output organization of the ventrolateral nucleus (VL) of the thalamus was analyzed electrophysiologically and morphologically at the single cell level. Virtually all pyramidal tract neurons in the motor cortex and area 6 received convergent inputs from the dentate (DN) and the interpositus (IN) nuclei and about 60% of thalamocortical (TC) neurons received convergent inputs from both the DN and the IN. Anterograde labelling following focal injection of *Phaseolus vulgaris* leukoagglutinin and intracellular staining of TC axons showed that the terminals in layer III tended to aggregate into patches about 1–1.5 mm wide in a frontal plane, which were arranged in longitudinal strips about 2–5 mm long in a rostrocaudal direction.

Introduction

The motor cortex receives one of its main inputs from the cerebellum through the ventrolateral nucleus (VL) of the thalamus [1–7]. In the previous studies, the responses of neurons in the motor cortex or thalamocortical (TC) neurons were elicited by stimulation of the brachium conjunctivum (BC). BC stimulation cannot provide information as to distinctive features of the projections of individual cerebellar nuclei to the motor cortex. Information relevant to projections of the separate cerebellar nuclei has been provided by two subsequent studies, using separate stimulation of the cerebellar nuclei combined with systematic mapping of the evoked potentials on the cortex [8, 9]. Both of these studies showed that the interpositus (IN) and the dentate nuclei

1011–6125/93/0603–0017 $ 2.75/0

(DN) project to the motor cortex (area 4) and area 6 [10]. Both studies were in agreement that both the IN and the DN projections in the motor cortex overlap considerably. This result suggests two possible neural organizations underlying the relation of cerebellar inputs and motor cortex outputs; single corticofugal neurons receive inputs from only one cerebellar nucleus and the neurons receiving inputs from separate cerebellar nuclei intermingle in a circumscribed area in the cortex, or all corticofugal neurons receive convergent inputs from more than one cerebellar nucleus. Since the study by Yoshida et al. [3], no detailed analyses of the neural circuits of the cerebello-cerebral connections had been reported using an intracellular recording method.

This paper will describe our recent data on the inputs from individual cerebellar nuclei to single TC neurons in the VL of the thalamus and single pyramidal tract neurons (PTNs) and other corticofugal neurons in the motor cortex and area 6 in the cat. In the second part of the paper, single cell morphology of neurons in the cerebello-thalamo-cortical pathway will be presented to provide morphological basis for the electrophysiologically determined neural circuitry.

Convergent Inputs from the Interpositus and the Dentate nuclei to PTNs in the Motor Cortex and Thalamocortical Neurons in the VL

In order to investigate connections between individual cerebellar nuclei and single cortical neurons, postsynaptic potentials were intracellularly recorded in the 'forelimb area' of the motor cortex and in the medial portion of the precruciate gyrus (area 6) [11].

Figure 1A–D shows an example of intracellular responses to stimulation of the VL and separate cerebellar nuclei in a single fast PTN. EPSPs were evoked from the VL at a latency of 1.3 ms (fig. 1B). Because of the short latency, they were considered to be monosynaptic [5, 12]. The lack of temporal facilitation with a pair of stimuli supported this conclusion [3, 13]. Stimulation of the onterpositus posterior (IP) evoked large, sharp-rising excitatory postsynaptic potentials (EPSPs) (fig. 1C.). DN stimulation also induced large EPSPs in the same neuron at approximately the same latency as IP stimulation (fig. 1D). As in this example, single PTNs, both fast and slow PTNs, in areas 4 and 6 received convergent inputs from both the IN and the DN. The percentage of the PTNs receiving convergent inputs from both the DN and the

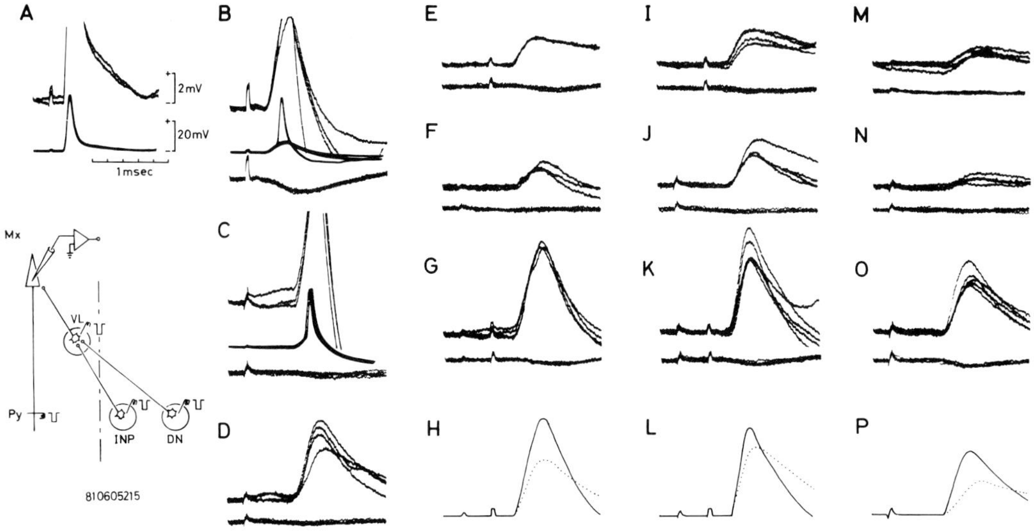

Fig. 1. Convergence of the interpositus and dentate inputs to single pyramidal tract neurons (**A–L**) and the convergent site of signals from both cerebellar nuclei in the cerebello-thalamo-cerebral pathway (**M–P**). **A** intracellular recording of antidromic spikes from a PTN in area 4 following medullary pyramid stimulation (stimulus intensity: 450 μA). **B** Ipsilateral VL stimulation produced short-latency EPSPs with some orthodromic spikes (250 μA). **C, D** Stimulation of the contralateral interpositus and dentate nuclei produced longer latency EPSPs with orthodromic spikes (**C,** 200 μA) and without spikes (**D,** 300 μA). **E, F** Stimulation of the VL (**E**) and the IP (**F**) at intensities slightly stronger than thresholds induced EPSPs with moderate amplitudes (**E,** 70 μA; **F,** 70 μA). **G** The stimuli of the VL and the IP with the same intensities as in **E** and **F** were delivered at such an interval that the onsets of the EPSPs evoked from two stimulus sites coincided in the PTN. **H** The amplitude of the EPSPs in G (solid line) was much larger than the algebraic sum of individual EPSPs evoked independently from the VL and the IP. **I–L** Similar to **E–H**, but the VL and the DN were stimulated (**I,** 70 μA; **J,** 250 μA). **M–P** Spatial facilitation of the interpositus and the dentate inputs. Stimulation of the IP (**M**) and the DN (**N**) at just above threshold produced small EPSPs in the same neuron (**M,** 60 μA; **N,** 200 μA). Simultaneous stimulation of the IP and the DN at the same intensities as in **M** and **N** induced large EPSPs in **O. P** The amplitude in **O** (solid line) was much larger than the algebraic sum of the EPSPs in **M** and **N** (dotted line). A lower trace in each record is an extracellular field potential taken after withdrawal. Schematic diagram of the experimental set-up and the presumed neural connections is shown on the left. From figure 7 in Shinoda et al. [11].

IN was about 85%, when PTNs were selected from the experiments in which at least two stimulating electrodes were placed in each nucleus [11, 14].

Besides PTNs, various corticofugal neurons in the motor cortex project to different subcortical nuclei. There had been no data available on the cerebellar inputs to corticofugal neurons in areas 4 and 6 projecting to different subcortical nuclei. There are two types of projections to the RN and the PN; projections by terminals of corticonuclear neurons proper, and by collaterals of corticofugal neurons sending their stem axons further down the brain stem. A substantial number of these various corticofugal neurons receive cerebellar inputs in areas 4 and 6 [15].

Since single PTNs received convergent inputs from both the DN and the IP, the question arose as to whether this convergence occurs at the level of the cortex or at the level of the VL. The site of convergence of the two inputs was determined by analysing the interaction between IP- and DN-evoked EPSPs. Figure 1M–P shows an example of an experiment in which the presence or absence of spatial facilitation between the DN and IP inputs was investigated. Stimulation of the IP and the DN evoked disynaptic EPSPs in the fast PTN (fig. 1M, N). Simultaneous stimulation of the IP and the DN at these intensities evoked EPSPs (fig. 10) larger than the algebraic sum (fig. 1P) of individual EPSPs evoked separately from the IP (fig. 1M) and the DN (fig. 1N), indicating that there was spatial facilitation at the last-order relay neurons in the pathways. Therefore, it was concluded that at least some convergence of the dentate and the interpositus inputs occurs at the level of the VL. In terms of cerebellar inputs to slow PTNs, the above method was not effective to determine the site of convergence, since the connection between the VL and slow PTNs was mostly disynaptic.

To confirm the above finding more directly, we recorded intracellular potentials from TC neurons in the VL and examined the effects of stimulation of both nuclei [16]. Figure 2B shows a typical example of inputs from the cerebellar nuclei to a TC neuron. TC neurons were identified by their antidromic responses to stimulation of the motor cortex (fig. 2A). Unitary EPSPs of different shapes were evoked in an all-or-none manner at threshold by stimulation of the IP (fig. 2B 1, 2) and the DN (fig. 2B 3, 4). Judging from the positions of the stimulating electrodes and the low stimulus intensities, we concluded that this TC neuron received convergent inputs from both the IP and the DN. A typical

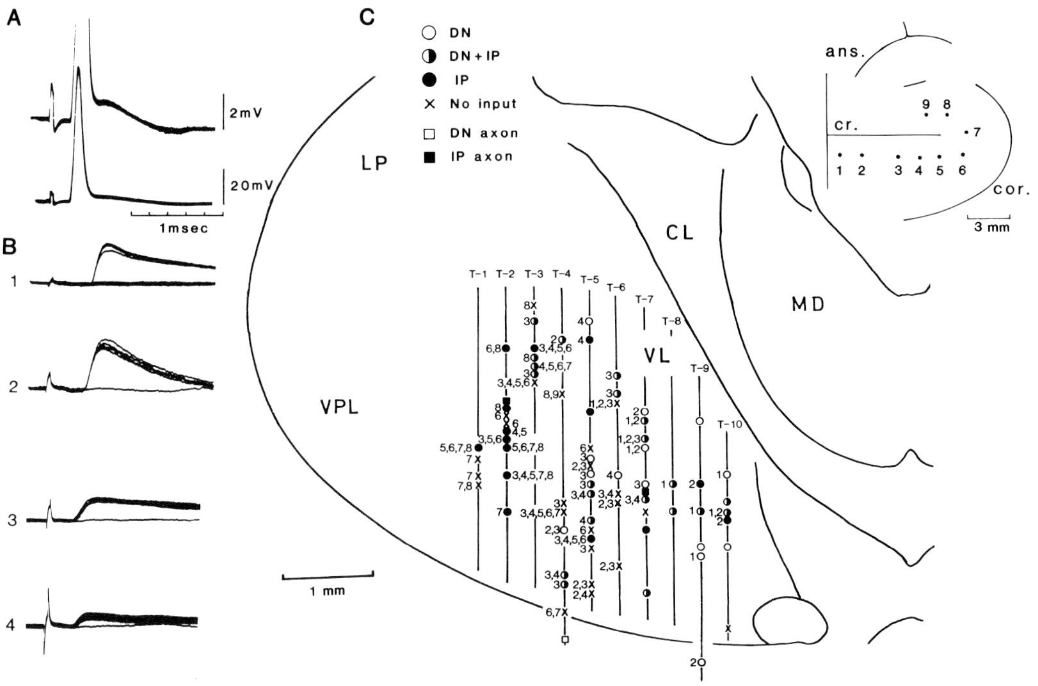

Fig. 2. Convergence of dentate and interpositus projections onto single thalamocortical neurons in the VL. **A** Antidromic response of a thalamocortical neuron evoked by stimulation of the motor cortex at suprathreshold. **B** Monosynaptic unitary EPSPs evoked in an all-or-none fashion from the interpositus (1, 2) and the dentate nucleus (3, 4) at thresholds with 110, 75, 70 and 80 μA, respectively. These EPSPs had different shapes and time courses. **C** Thalamic distribution of thalamocortical neurons receiving inputs from the interpositus and the dentate nuclei. Seventy-three cells and three axons were penetrated intracellularly, using a single micropipette throughout the experiment. Mapping was done systematically at 300-μm intervals lateromedially at the same frontal plane of the thalamus (10.0 mm anterior to the ear bar position). The electrode was advanced dorsoventrally in one direction and was not pulled back until the ventral margin of the thalamus was reached. Circles = Neurons receiving inputs as indicated; crosses = neurons in which PSPs could not be evoked from either nucleus. Numbers in **C** indicate stimulating sites in the motorcortex for antidromic activation (see inset on the topright). From figures 1 and 7 in Shinoda et al. [11].

example of the distribution of inputs from the IP and the DN onto single TC neurons is shown in figure 2C. In this example, 73 TC neurons were recorded in the same frontal plane of the VL in the same cat, using the same microelectrode. Twenty-one of 50 neurons receiving cerebellar inputs (42%) received convergent inputs from both the DN and the IP. Some cells in the medial portion of the VL received mainly from the DN, some in the lateral portion of the VL mainly from the IP. The thalamic projection areas of the DN and the IP were wide and there was considerable overlap between the dentate and the interpositus projection areas in the VL. And in this overlapping area a considerable number of TC neurons received convergent inputs from both the DN and the IP. Out of 194 TC neurons recorded in the VL, 97 neurons (50%) had convergent inputs from the IP and DN. This percentage of the TC neurons receiving convergent inputs must be very much underestimated, since we could not activate all neurons in the IP or the DN without spread of the current to neurons in the other nucleus due to the small number of implanted stimulating electrodes and weak stimulus intensities. Similar results were also obtained by Rispal-Padel et al. [17]. These physiological findings are in agreement with the anatomical description of cerebellar projections to the VL [18, 19].

Fig. 3. Distribution of terminals of thalamocortical fibers originating from the ventrolateral nucleus of the thalamus. Right: Camera lucida drawing of PHA-L-labelled TC axons in the motor cortex. This drawing was made on a single frontal section (100 μm thick) and the location of this patch of axon terminals is shown in the inset on the bottom right. Cells in layer V are large pyramidal cells. The broken line on the bottom shows the border between the cortical gray and white matter. Roman letters show cortical layers. The injection site of PHA-L in the VA-VL complex is shown on the bottom left. Cru = cruciate sulcus; presyl = presylvian sulcus; VA = ventroanterior nucleus; VM = ventromedial nucleus; AV = anteroventral nucleus; VL = ventrolateral nucleus. Left: Two longitudinal strips of labelled TC fibers in the motor cortex. Representative sections (100 μm thick) are separated by 600 μm. Note the terminal free gap between two patches that are arranged in a rostrocaudal direction. From figures 1 and 2 in Shinoda and Kakei [20].

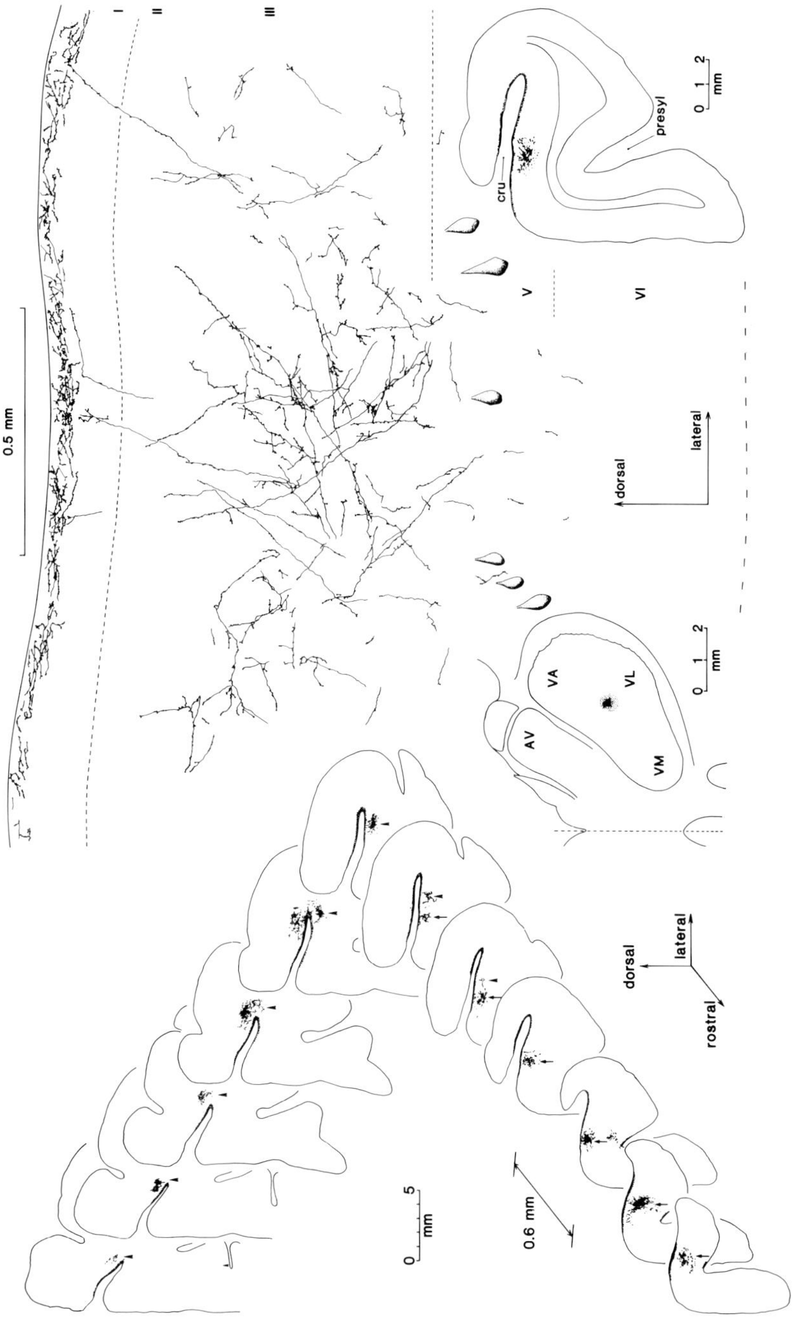
0.5 mm
I
II
III
V
VI
cru
presyl
0 1 2
mm
dorsal
lateral
VA
VL
AV
VM
0 1 2
mm
dorsal
lateral
rostral
0 5
mm
0.6 mm

3

Morphological Analysis of Thalamocortical Projection

The intracortical organization of TC fibers has been analyzed extensively in the visual system, but much less is known about the TC projection from the VL to the motor cortex. Therefore, we report the results of the experiments undertaken to visualize the three-dimensional distribution pattern of TC terminals and the morphology of single TC axons in the motor cortex, using the anterograde labelling method with *Phaseolus vulgaris* leukoagglutinin (PHA-L) and intracellular injection of horseradish peroxidase (HRP).

Anterograde labelling following focal injections of PHA-L was used to identify the three-dimensional cortical distribution of TC fibers in the motor cortex of the cat [20]. Iontophoretic injection of PHA-L resulted in well-localized injection sites (inset at the bottom of fig. 3). The injection sites were usually less than 1.0 mm, and sometimes as small as 400 μm in diameter. The morphology of the labelled fine axons, boutons en passant and various terminal specializations could be resolved (fig. 3), but the labelled structures had a more dusty appearance than those visualized by intracellular injection of HRP [21]. Fine axons and swellings en passant were found usually in cortical layers I and III (fig. 3), but in some animals, these were restricted to layer I or to layer III. Labelling of parent axons in the subcortical white matter was not observed.

Labelling of fine collaterals and swellings en passant in layer III was well localized in a mediolateral direction, and labelled fibers were grouped into discrete patches about 1–1.5 mm wide within layer III of the motor cortex. In contrast, when labelling appeared in layer I or in both layers I and III, labelled fibers in layer I were not confined mediolaterally within the same vertical band as the patches in layer III, but rather extended widely in a mediolateral direction beyond the area of the patches in layer III. To determine the pattern in which the patches of the labelled fibers were organized over a wide cortical area, we attempted to reconstruct patches from serial sections. In this reconstruction, it turned out that patches of the labelled fibers about 1–1.5 mm wide on individual sections were aligned in a rostrocaudal direction, making a longitudinal strip as viewed from the surface. In representative frontal sections at 600-μm intervals (fig. 3, left), the patches indicated by upward arrows continued on into the ventral bank of the cruciate sulcus, more or less in parallel to a sagittal plane in a rostrocaudal direction over a distance of 3.8 mm. Longitudinal strips ranged from 2 to 5 mm in length (n = 6). Their location was almost in parallel to a sagittal plane, but the strips ran slightly obliquely, rostromedially to caudolaterally. A small focal injection in the VA-VL complex usually resulted in multiple strips of labelled fibers in the motor cortex. The number of longitudinal strips varied, depending on the amount of PHA-L injected. Two to 7 strips were differentiated in 4 cats. Roughly parallel strips, each about 1–1.5 mm wide, were separated from each other by regions in which the label was much diminished or practically absent.

Morphology of Single Thalamocortical Axons in the Motor Cortex

During the electrophysiological experiments described before, we found that about 40% of TC neurons were antidromically activated from three or more sites in the motor cortex separated from each other by 1.5–2 mm, indicating the single TC neurons project to multiple zones in the motor cortex (fig. 2C) [16]. The projection of single TC axons to multiple foci was further investigated morphologically by intraaxonal injection of HRP into physiologically identified TC axons. The intracortical trajectory of single axons of TC neurons receiving monosynaptic inputs from the cerebellar nuclei was reconstructed three-dimensionally on serial sections.

The typical branching pattern of a single TC axon in the motor cortex is shown in figure 4. TC axons originating from the VA-VL complex divided into several main branches in the white matter below the gray matter. They further divided into numerous branches, forming multiple plexuses of terminals in the cerebral gray matter, mainly in layer III and very rarely in layers I and VI. Each TC axon had 2–6 plexuses with an average diameter of 0.5 mm. These plexuses of single TC axons were separated by terminal-free gaps and distributed mainly in a rostrocaudal direction for a distance of up to 6 mm in the motor cortex. In a TC axon (fig. 4), terminals were distributed over a distance of 5.0 mm rostrocaudally and 4.8 mm mediolaterally in the forelimb area of the motor cortex. At least 5 plexuses were identified in this axon, although four of them overlapped in the lateral view. This rostrocaudal extension of single TC axons fits well with the rostrocaudal strips of TC axon terminals observed with PHA-L (fig. 3). Axon terminals of TC neurons were distributed in both layers I and III in the motor cortex in PHA-L experiments. Single axon staining with HRP, however, showed that axon terminals were mainly distributed in layer III. This discrepancy of the two results probably suggests that there are at least two different types of TC neurons; one projecting to layer III and the other projecting to layer I, and further suggests that the latter TC neurons must have finer axons, since we could not penetrate those axons with a glass microelectrode in a good condition. Taking this morphology of single TC axons into account, the result obtained with the PHA-L labelling method implies that a cluster of TC neurons in a focal area of the VA-VL complex, each with projection distributed over wide rostrocaudal region of the cortex, make up the longitudinal strips of axon terminals. The extent of single plexuses of TC axon terminals almost corresponds to the size of individual motor efferent columns or zones defined by intracortical microstimulation [22].

Discussion

The present finding of the cortical distribution of TC axons from the VA-VL complex is in agreement with that of Strick and Sterling [23] in that terminals are distributed mainly in layers I and III. Sasaki et al. [24] suggested from the electrophysiological study that there should be superficial and deep TC projections. These dual projections were demonstrated anatomically [25, 26]. More recently, Jinnai et al. [27] reported that TC neurons in the VA-VL complex which receive inputs from the globus pallidus, but not from the cerebellar nuclei, project to layer I of the anterior sigmoid gyrus in the cat. However, a focal injection of PHA-L in the caudal portion of the VA-VL complex where

---

Fig. 4. Axonal branches of a single thalamocortical neuron in the motor cortex of the cat. Lateral view of the branches in the lateral portion of the pericruciate cortex. The mediolateral extension of axon terminals of this axon in 4,800 μm. This axon, penetrated in the cerebral white matter (indicated by an arrow), was activated directly from the ipsilateral VL and monosynaptically from the contralateral cerebellar nucleus. From figure 2 in Shinoda et al. [31].

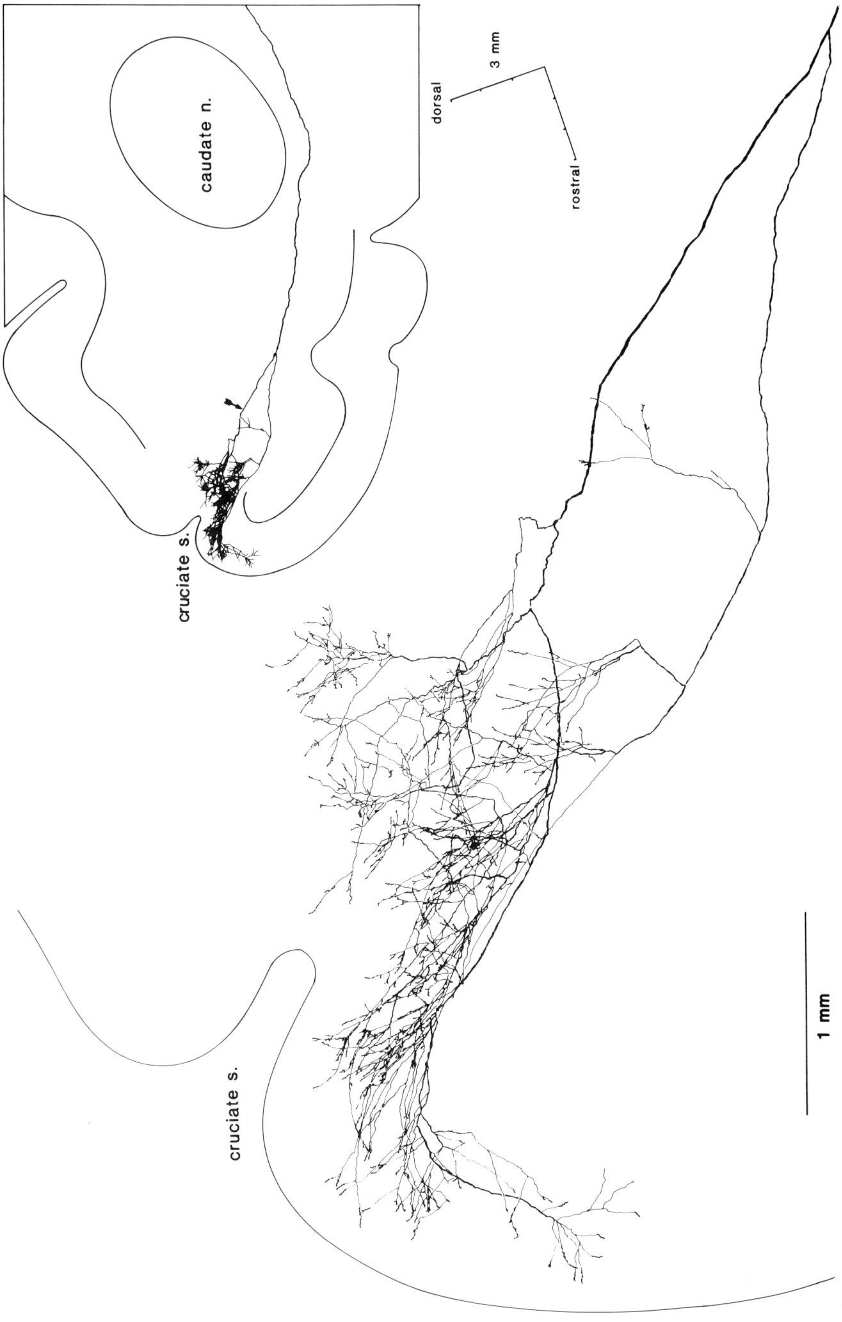

4

the cerebellar projection exists resulted in labelling of TC fibers in both layers I and III in the present study. This discrepancy remains unresolved. One possibility is that small neurons projecting only to layer I may be involved in the caudal part of the VA-VL complex [25].

The functional significance of the convergent inputs from the DN and the IP can be appreciated by reviewing the previous studies on the role of the lateral cerebellum, which projects primarily via the DN, as contrasted to the role of the intermediate zone of the cerebellar cortex, which projects primarily via the IN. The lateral cerebellum receives inputs mainly from the cerebral 'association cortex', while the pars intermedia of the cerebellum receives inputs mainly from the sensorymotor cortex and also from the periphery. It has been proposed that the dentate output which receives input from certain parts of the cerebral 'association cortex' plays a role in initiating PTN activity in the motor cortex prior to movement, and that, with onset of movement, the IN receives the pyramidal tract signals representing the motor command, and a spinal input that provides a feedback signal via the pars intermedia, so that PTNs receiving these signals via the thalamus may perform corrections of movements [4, 6, 28, 29]. If the IN and the DN had differential projections to the different regions of the motor cortex, the above-mentioned signals including different informations from the IN and the DN would exert their separate influences on PTNs innervating muscles of different body parts. On the other hand, if the IN and DN projected to different PTNs in a circumscribed area of the motor cortex, separate input-output lines would exist and differential activities of PTNs would result. But the present study has demonstrated that the signals from the IN and DN converge on the majority of single PTNs and other corticofugal neurons in the 'forelimb area' of the motor cortex and area 6, although some regional difference exists for the relative strength of the respective inputs. In this respect, the present finding favors the generally believed concept that single PTNs are common paths leading out of the cortex.

The importance of cerebrocerebellar interactions for control of movement was proposed by Evarts and Thach [4] and later this notion was further elaborated on the programming and execution of voluntary movement by Allen and Tsukahara [6]. The cerebro-cerebello-cerebral loop was assumed to exist between the cerebral cortex and the cerebellar hemisphere on the basis of the field potential analysis by Sasaki [30]. The present study confirmed the existence of the cerebro-cerebellar loop and further demonstrated the existence of the excitatory feedback loop between the cerebral cortex and the cerebellar nuclei at the single-cell level. Cortical outputs from area 6 are all excitatory and are conveyed to the pontine nuclei mainly by CPNs and partly by collaterals of PTNs, and also to other precerebellar nuclei such as the nucleus reticularis tegmenti pontis and the inferior olive. The neurons in these nuclei, in turn, exert their excitatory influence on the DN [31]. Then, the excitatory output from the DN is fed back to CPNs and PTNs in areas 4 and 6 by way of the VL [11, 16]. On the other hand, cortical outputs from area 4 are conveyed to the pontine nuclei mainly by axon collaterals of PTNs and partly by CPNs and also to other precerebellar nuclei such as the inferior olive and lateral reticular nucleus. The neurons receiving input from area 4 in these precerebellar nuclei exert excitatory effects on the IN. Then, the output from the IN is fed back mainly to PTNs and CPNs in area 4 and less strongly to those in area 6 by way of the VL. The cerebellar cortex also receives the same input from the corresponding cerebral cortex and sends out signals to the underlying cerebellar nucleus, so that the excitatory inputs to the cerebellar nuclei are modulated spatially and temporally and are converted into the organized output of signals that results in finely controlled movement. In addition to the cerebro-cerebello-cerebral pathways, two more cortico-subcortico-cortical pathways exist; cortico-thalamo-cortical and cortico-striopallido-cortical pathways [6, 30, 32]. To gain a further insight into the manner in which the cerebrocerebellar excitatory loop receives its instructions and issues its own motor commands, we will need more information as to what signals are transmitted in these different loops, and how and where they interact to establish and maintain the intended motor set.

References

1 Cohen B, Housepian EM, Purpura DP: Intrathalamic regulation of activity in a cerebellocortical projection pathway. Exp Neurol 1962;6:492–506.

2 Frigyresi TL, Purpura DP: Functional properties of synaptic pathways influencing transmission in the specific cerebello-thalamocortical projection system. Exp Neurol 1964;10:305–324.

3 Yoshida M, Yajima K, Uno M: Different activation of the two types of pyramidal tract neurons through the cerebellothalamo-cortical pathway. Experientia 1966; 22:331–332.

4 Evarts EV, Thach WT; Motor mechanisms of the CNS: Cerebrocerebellar interactions. Ann Rev Physiol 1969;31:451–498.
5 Uno M, Yoshida M, Hirota I: The mode of cerebello-thalamic relay transmission investigated with intracellular recording from cells of the ventrolateral nucleus of cat's thalamus. Exp Brain Res 1970;10:121–139.
6 Allen GI, Tsukahara N: Cerebrocerebellar communication systems. Physiol Rev 1975;54:957–1006.
7 Rispal-Padel L, Grangetto A: The cerebello-thalamo-cortical pathway. Topographical investigation at the unitary level in the cat. Exp Brain Res 1977;28:101–123.
8 Sasaki K, Matsuda Y, Mizuno N: Distribution of cerebellar-induced responses in the cerebral cortex. Exp Neurol 1973;39:342–354.
9 Rispal-Padel L, Latreille J: The organization of projections from the cerebellar nuclei to the contralateral motor cortex in the cat. Exp Brain Res 1974;19: 36–60.
10 Hassler WR, Muhs-Clement K: Architektonischer Aufbau des sensorimotorischen und parietalen Cortex der Katze. J Hirnforsch 1964;6:377–420.
11 Shinoda Y, Kano M, Futami T: Synaptic organization of the cerebello-thalamo-cerebral pathway in the cat. I. Projection of individual cerebellar nuclei to single pyramidal tract neurons in areas 4 and 6. Neuroscience Res 1985;2:133–156.
12 Ammassian VE, Weiner H: Monosynaptic and polysynaptic activation of pyramidal tract neurons by thalamic stimulation; in Purpura DP, Yahr MD (eds): The Thalamus. New York, Columbia University Press, 1966, pp 255–286.
13 Deschênes M, Landry P, Clercq M: A reanalysis of the ventrolateral input in slow and fast pyramidal tract neurons of the cat motor cortex. Neuroscience 1982;7: 2149–2157.
14 Shinoda Y, Yamazaki M, Futami T: Convergent inputs from the dentate and the interpositus nuclei to pyramidal tract neurons in the motor cortex. Neurosci Lett 1982;34:111–115.
15 Futami T, Kano M, Sento S, Shinoda Y: Synaptic organization of the cerebello-thalamo-cerebral pathway in the cat. III. Cerebellar input to corticofugal neurons destined for different subcortical nuclei in areas 4 and 6. Neurosci Res 1986;3: 321–344.
16 Shinoda Y, Futami T, Kano M: Synaptic organization of the cerebello-thalamo-cerebral pathway in the cat. II. Input-output organization of single thalamocortical neurons in the ventrolateral thalamus. Neurosci Res 1985;2:157–180.
17 Rispal-Padel L, Troiani D, Harnois C: Converging cerebellofugal inputs to the thalamus. II. Analysis and topography of thalamic EPSPs induced by convergent monosynaptic interpositus and dentate inputs. Exp Brain Res 1989;68:59–72.
18 Angaut P: The cerebello-thalamic projections in the cat; in Massion J, Sasaki K (eds): Cerebro-Cerebellar Interactions. Amsterdam, Elsevier, 1979, pp 19–43.
19 Sugimoto T, Mizuno N. Itoh K: An autoradiographic study on the terminal distribution of cerebellothalamic fibers in the cat. Brain Res 1981;215:29–47.
20 Shinoda Y, Kakei S: Distribution of terminals of thalamocortical fibers originating from the ventrolateral nucleus of the cat thalamus. Neurosci Lett 1989;96:163–167.
21 Shinoda Y: General Discussion 3; in: Motor Areas of the Cerebral Cortex, Ciba Foundation Symposium, 132. New York, Wiley, 1987, pp 221–230.

22 Asanuma H, Sakata H: Functional organization of a cortical efferent system examined with focal depth stimulation in cats. J Neurophysiol 1967;30:35–54.
23 Strick PL, Sterling P: Synaptic termination of afferents from the ventrolateral nucleus of the thalamus in the cat motor cortex. A light and electron microscope study. J Comp Neurol 1974;153:77–106.
24 Sasaki K, Stanton HP, Dieckman G: Characteristic features of augmenting and recruiting responses in the cerebral cortex. Exp Neurol 1970;26:369–392.
25 Penny GR, Itoh K, Diamond II: Cells of different sizes in the ventral nuclei project to different layers of the somatic cortex in the cat. Brain Res 1982;242:55–65.
26 Kawaguchi S, Samejima A, Yamamoto T: Post-natal development of the cerebello-cerebral projection in kittens. J Physiol (Lond) 1983;343:215–232.
27 Jinnai K, Nambu A, Yoshida S: Thalamic afferents to layer I of anterior sigmoid cortex originating from the VA-VL neurons with entopeduncular input. Exp Brain Res 1987;69:67–76.
28 Massion J, Sasaki K: Cerebro-Cerebellar Interactions. Amsterdam, Elsevier, 1979.
29 Brooks VB, Thach WT: Cerebellar control of posture and movement; in Brookhart JM, Mountcastle VB (eds): Handbook of Physiology. The Nervous System, vol II, part 2, 1981, pp 877–946.
30 Sasaki K: Cerebro-cerebellar interconnections in cats and monkeys; in Massion J, Sasaki K (eds): Cerebro-Cerebellar Interactions. Amsterdam, Elsevier, 1979, pp 105–124.
31 Shinoda Y, Sugiuchi Y, Futami T: Excitatory inputs to cerebellar dentate nucleus neurons from the cerebral cortex in the cat. Exp Brain Res 1987;67:299–315.
32 Evarts EV, Shinoda Y, Wise S: Neurophysiological Approaches in Higher Brain Functions. New York, Wiley, 1984, pp 91–126.

Dr. Yoshikazu Shinoda, MD, Department of Physiology,
School of Medicine Tokyo Medical and Dental University, Tokyo (Japan)

Proceedings of the 2nd International Workshop on Microphysiological Recordings during Stereotactic Neurosurgery: Motor Thalamus, October 1–2, 1989, Nikko, Japan
Stereotact Funct Neurosurg 1993;60:32–41

The Primate Motor Thalamus Analysed with Reference to Subcortical Afferent Territories

G. Percheron, C. François, B. Talbi, J.F. Meder, G. Fenelon, J. Yelnik

Laboratoire de neuromorphologie informationnelle et de neurologie expérimentale du mouvement, Pavillon Inserm, Hôpital de la Salpêtrière, Paris, France

Key Words. Thalamus · Motor system · Basal ganglia · Primates

Abstract. This paper analyses the internal organisation of the primate motor thalamus. A topographic study of the three main subcortical afferent territories (the cerebellar, pallidal and nigral territories) gives a much simpler and more functionally relevant partitioning of the thalamus than consideration of conflictual cytoarchitectonic nuclei.

One of the main difficulties in understanding the internal organisation of the thalamus stems from the limits of the few conceptual tools that have been used for its analysis. The thalamus is currently conceived as a conglomeration of 'nuclei' with different 'pars'. These continue to be given the attributes of the historical 'centres' [1], namely each centre occupies a definite portion of space limited by a regular wall, the content of the box is homogeneous and characteristic of each centre, the source and morphology of afferent axons and the cerebral targets are particular to each centre. According to the associationist interpretation (and its 'box-and-arrow diagram'), each centre contains a 'function' which is determined by its connections. Sensory 'relays' such as the lateral geniculate body mostly comply with the assumed properties just mentioned. This is not the case with the motor thalamus. The variety of boundaries and labels found in the literature is a reason for being wary about the assumptions concerning 'thalamic nuclei'. For historical reasons, partly linked to the available histological techniques, the thalamic centre is nowadays essentially a 'cytoarchitectonic nucleus'. This is only one among several distinct neuronal set spaces [1] occupied only by the somata of neurons (fig. 1), Dendritic arboriza-

1011–6125/93/0603–0032 $ 2.75/0

tions, by far the most important part for information reception, often cross the 'somatic border', which accounts for the fact that neurons can be influenced by information arriving outside this border. The informationally significant boundary is the 'dendritic border', containing all the dendritic arborizations of the same neuronal species defined as the set made up of the neurons which have statistically similar dendritic arborizations. The corresponding space is called a 'patria' (or dendritic land). The space occupied by the dendritic arborizations of similar neurons of one patria projecting to the same target is termed a 'source space'. The space occupied by all the axonal endings, or 'cladons', from one source is termed a territory, with a 'cladonal border'. The claim that a thalamic nucleus, always and perfectly, realises the coincidence of emission, reception and communication spaces, i.e. dendritic lands, source spaces, territories and domains, is in most cases fallacious. Precise cartographic studies of the motor thalamus demonstrate that such a coincidence must not be taken for granted but carefully verified each time. In addition to tracing methods, Golgi studies reconstructing entire neuronal arborescences are necessary. The motor thalamus is made up of about 75% of 'tufted neurons' and of local circuit 'microneurones'. Since Mannen [2], it has become important to determine how dendritic arborizations participate in the closure of 'nuclei'. Some nuclei, such as the lateral geniculate and the anterior nuclei, are enclosed within a wall made up of myelinated fibers that thalamic dendrites do not cross (enclosed patriae, fig. 1A). This wall separates an inside from an outside and facilitates observation of the coincidence with the border of an afferent territory. There is another case of obvious closure which can be discerned only in Golgi material. This is when, without any fibrous capsule, the dendrites of two neighbouring patriae bend along a common barrier that they do not cross (insulated patriae, fig. 1B). This can be observed for instance between the pulvinar and the somesthetic nucleus. But the separation between motor thalamic nuclei is still different. There is no wall, and no bending of the dendrites. One pattern is particularly characeristic. A 'spacing strip' separates the somata of two adjacent patriae at a distance such that their (short) dendrites do not intermingle. This has cytoarchitectonic manifestation: a strip with few or no cells (fig. 1C). There is another case with no cytoarchitectonic sign. The separation between two neighbouring thalamic regions with intertwined dendritic arborizations is only effectuated by the spatial segregation of the two adjacent afferent terri-

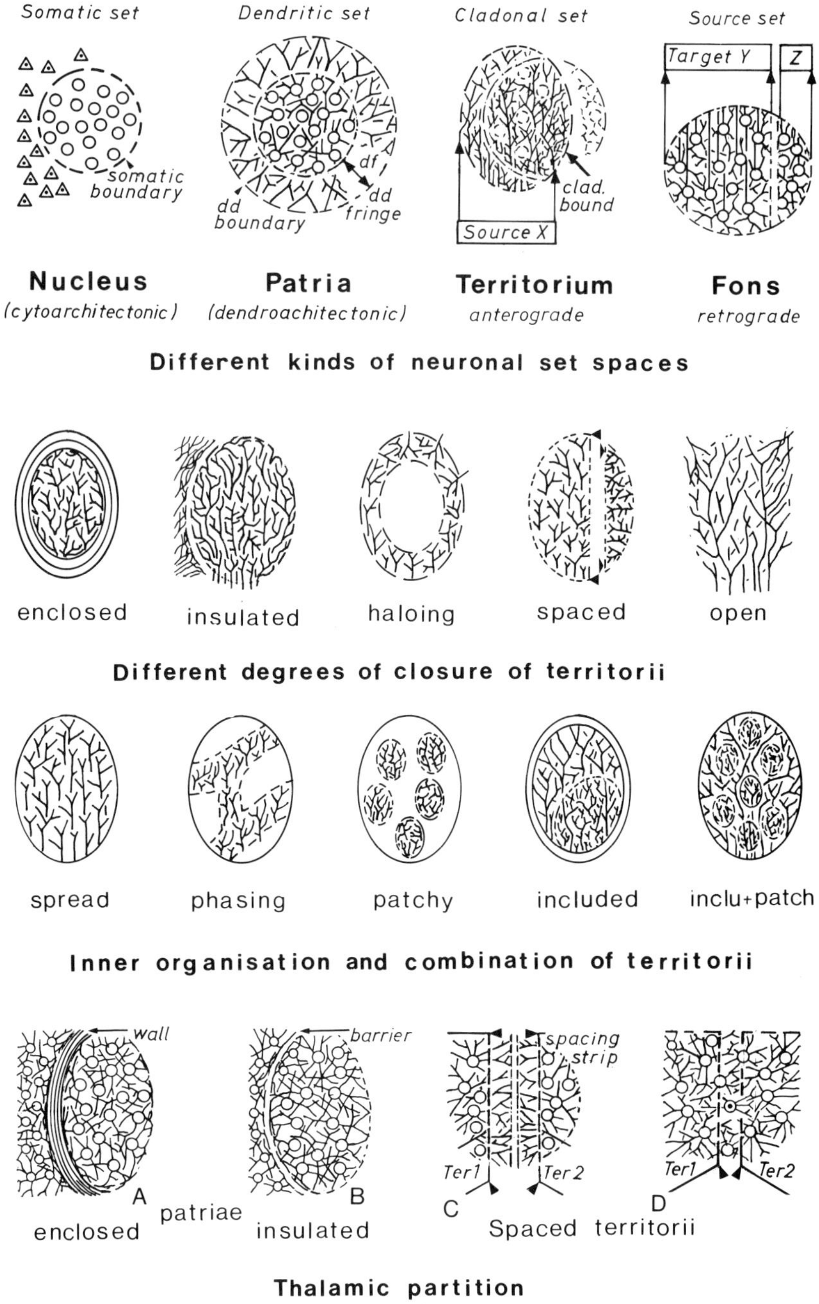

Fig. 1. Theoretical neuronal set spaces.

tories, the cladons of which do not intermingle (fig. 1D). The most fruitful recent advance in the understanding of the motor thalamus has been the general recognition that the easiest way of analysing its inner organisation is the topographic description of its subcortical afferent territories. The internal organisation of these territories is not always homogeneous. The spatial distribution of territories from different sources can have different combinatory modalities. They can overlap totally or partially. Patchy or sparse territories may be included within another continuous dense 'master territory' (fig. 1).

Our material was obtained from 20 macaques from 3 species (*Macaca mulatta, fascicularis* and *nemestrina*) and was made up of 8 cerebellectomies, 1 cerebellar, 5 pallidal and 6 nigral stereotactic injections of tritiated amino acids. The histological techniques used were Wiitanen's techniques and autoradiography. The three-dimensional geometry of these territories is so complex that reconstructions from topographic data obtained from closely spaced regular sections located according to a precise cartographic system of coordinates are absolutely necessary. This system, in our material, is always the same, i.e. that based on the two commissural points CA and CP [3]. Such a cartographic method made possible the comparison from one individual to another and three-dimensional analyses.

Description of the primate motor thalamus raises a first fundamental question. Is the primate motor thalamus a separate entity? A comparison between the respective topographies of the territories from the dorsal column nuclei and from the cerebellum in chimpanzees [4] and in Macaques (5, 6] clearly showed that they indeed constitute separate territories. An obvious cytoarchitectonic spacing strip located between VCL (VCe, VPLc or VPL) and VIL (VIme or VPLo) represents a sort of intrathalamic Rolando sulcus separating the motor thalamus from the somatosensory territory. The latter is the territory occupied by the cladons from the dorsal column nuclei, from the trigeminal complex and by the bulk of the spinothalamic cladons. The separation between the somatosensory and the motor thalamus has been recently obscured by the controversy over the exact location of the territory of the cladons conveying proprioceptive ('deep' or musculo-articular) messages. It has been repeatedly observed in humans as well as in monkeys that such messages are systematically separated from cutaneous ones and are always located more anteriorly and more dorsally. Two contradictory interpretations have been opposed [7]: that of Ohye et al. [8], according to which the topography of deep messages corresponds to a part of the cerebellar territory where tremorosynchronous activity is recorded (the 'Vim'), and that of Lenz et al. [9], according to which deep messages are conversely located in an 'anterior part' of the lemnical territory. Two recent papers [7, 10] strongly support the second hypothesis. Our preliminary topographic study in humans and our experimental work in macaques seem to be in favour of the former. This particular problem will be left for future investigation.

Our description of the primate motor thalamus with reference to subcortical afferent territories starts in front of the lemniscal territory and goes progressively from caudal to rostral. It will successively cover three main territories: the cerebellar, pallidal and nigral territories. The cerebellar territory is primarily that which is occupied by the cladons from the dentate nucleus. Axons of cerebellar origin constitute the brachium conjunctivum. After decussation they run through or go round the nucleus ruber and arrive in the ventral part of the thalamus, where they fan out. The cerebellar territory is very dense. Its three-dimensional geometry is complex. In a sagittal reconstruction it is banana-shaped with a marked anterior convexity. Its posterior part is purely dorsal and is made up of a lateral and a medial extension. The former fades out progressively in the superolateral corner of the lateral mass. The latter is located within the dorsal extension of the lamina medullaris interna. More anteriorly the cerebellar territory extends continuously from the dorsal part of the lateral mass to the paralaminar part of the medial complex. Still more anteriorly the cerebellar territory slopes down, becoming very large and extending over the whole width of the lateral mass. In its anterior portion, the posterior part of the pallidal territory causes it to separate into two parts, one medial and one lateral, which pull away from each other progressively. The cerebellar territory ends anteriorly in the form of small medial and lateral islands. A comparison of the three-dimensional distribution of the territory with cytoarchitectonic pictures shows that it corresponds to several cytoarchitectonic nuclei. Only a single ventral nucleus, the VIL (VIme or VPLo), with its large sparsely distributed somata, is easily recognisable. The VIM (VImi or area X) is less characteristic. In the dorsal nuclei, it is very difficult to identify, by cytoarchitectonic means alone, the place where cerebellar axons end. In addition to cladons from dentate origin, the cerebellar territory is also occupied by cladons from the two interpositi nuclei and from the fastigial nuclei. The fastigial territory is patchy and included in the posterior and dorsal part of the cerebellar territory, particularly in the portion which overhangs the lemniscal territory. The cerebellar territory still includes sparse islands of cladons from the vestibular complex and from spino-thalamic neurons.

Before our first precise cartographic work [11, 12], it was generally believed in animals including monkeys that there was a single motor nucleus, the so-called VL nucleus, receiving confluent afferents from the cerebellum and from the pallidum. It is now accepted that there is in fact a complete separation between the two territories, effectuated by means of a clearly visible spacing strip. The pallidal territory is located in front of the cerebellar territory. Pallidal axons constitute the ansa lenticularis [13], cross through the internal capsule, make up the V-shaped Forel's 'fields' (H2, H and H1) and arrive at the ventral border of the thalamus from where they fan out in front of the cerebellar axons. The pallidal territory is intensively but inhomogeneously dense. Dorsolaterally directed oblique oblong patches receiving more numerous pallidal cladons can be observed. The three-dimensional geometry of the territory is complex. It appears as banana-shaped after sagittal reconstruction with the same curvature as that of the cerebellar territory as it is also in transverse section, where its lateral convexity follows that of the lateral border of the thalamus. Caudally, the pallidal territory is dorsal, being above the cerebellar territory. More anteriorly it progressively slopes down and separates the cerebellar territory into its medial and lateral anterior extensions. Anteriorwards it expands progressively. It covers the whole ventrocaudal extent of the lateral mass of the thalamus of which it occupies a little more than its lateral half. This width progressively decreases anteriorwards. The pallidal territory ends along the lateral border just before reaching the anterior pole of the thalamus. The pallidal territory also corresponds to several cytoarchitectonic nuclei. Only the cloud-shaped ventral nucleus (VOL, VOe or VLo), with its smaller and paler neurons, is distinctive [12]. Denser oblong islands correspond to the denser patches of pallidal cladons. The dorsal part of the territory does not coincide with clearly delineated cytoarchitectonic nuclei; the border of DO (DOe or posterodorsal part of VA) cannot be traced using purely cytoarchitectonic criteria. The pallidal territory within the centre median complex although it is an authentic part of the motor thalamus [14] will not be considered in the present account.

The nigral territory was not recognised in Hassler's two atlases [15,

16] and even now is often undervaluated [10, 17]. The nigral territory nevertheless is another major subcortical afferent to the motor thalamus. In the monkey, it is located in front of the cerebellar territory, from which it is clearly separated [18], and medial to the pallidal territory, from which it is also topographically distinct [19]. The separation between the latter two is effectuated simply by the segregation of the cladons without any visible spacing strip. Axons from the pars reticulata and from the pars mixta of the substantia nigra are gathered together medially and then lead upwards in the vicinity of the mammillo-thalamic tract. They reach the thalamus ventrally, medial to the pallidal axons. The nigral territory is dense with a decreasing density from medial to lateral. Its three-dimensional geometry is complex. Its caudal part is located in the ventral and medial portion of the lateral mass just in front of the centre median complex and, also, continuously through the lamina, in the paralaminar region of the medial complex. More anteriorly, the nigral territory surrounds the mammillo-thalamic tract and covers the whole ventrodorsal extent of the lateral mass of the thalamus. The topography of the nigral territory also corresponds to several cytoarchitectonic nuclei [18]: the LPo (VA anterior) and VOM (Voi or Vamc and other parts of VA) nuclei, the anterior paralaminar part of the medial complex (MDmf), and islands in the medial nucleus (M, or MDpc). There is still controversy [8, 17, 18] over the existence of a territory in front of the pallidal and nigral territories, which affects the definition and acceptance of a VA or lateral polar nucleus. Work in progress is providing evidence that the pallidal and nigral territories entirely fill this pole.

The motor thalamus can thus very simply be described as being composed of 3 main subcortical afferent territories; one depending on the cerebellum and the two others on the basal ganglia. Figure 2 shows that, in comparison to this plan, even if nuclei and territories are not equivalent and therefore should not be forced to coincide, the various nomenclatures used for the description of cytoarchitectonic nuclei [10, 12, 17, 18, 21–28] are conflicting. The recent progress in the cartography of the subcortical afferents in the monkey motor thalamus has shown that, except at some well-known precise locations, cytoarchitectonics is of limited value in isolating functionally relevant thalamic parts. Even the historical partitioning into ventral and dorsal cytoarchitectonic nuclei (fig. 2) appears to have no foundation with regards to the distribution of the subcortical afferents. Conversely, consideration of subcorti-

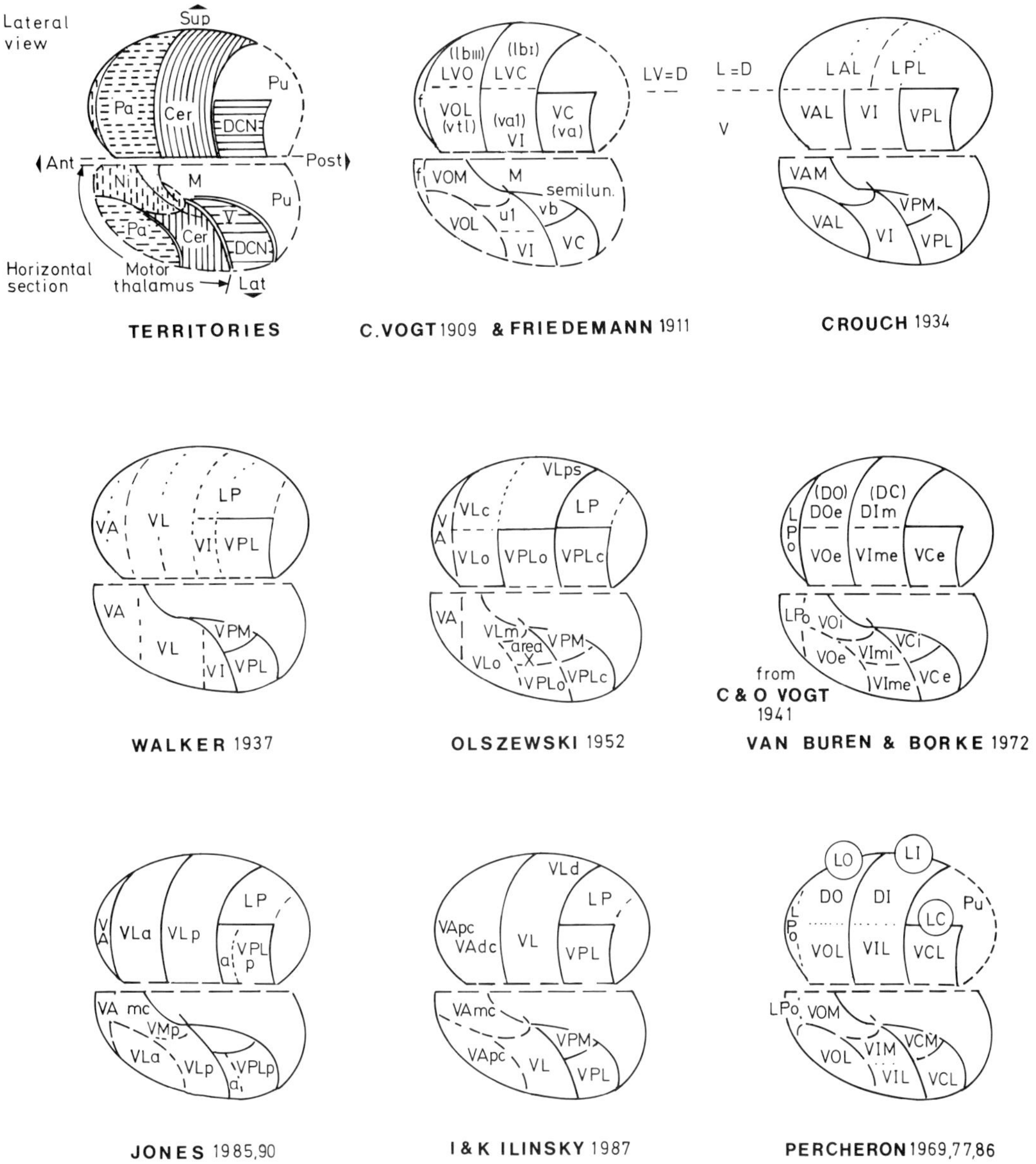

Fig. 2. Schematic topographic distribution of the afferent subcortical territories in the primate motor thalamus and some of the cytoarchitectonic partitions from the literature.

cal territories has a strong systemic meaning, suppresses cultural conflicts about nomenclature and greatly simplifies the partitioning of the motor thalamus.

The fact that it is not possible to delineate directly subcortical territories in the human motor thalamus is highly detrimental to its understanding and to the therapy that might be offered to patients. There is, however, some hope that, in addition to indirect cytoarchitectonic signs such as the tracing of spacing strips, immunocytochemistry will enable the transfer of experimental data obtained in monkeys for the partitioning of the human thalamus into territories [7, 10, 29]. Among other expected advantages, the delimitation of territories of afferents, instead of nuclei, within the human motor thalamus could lead to the isolation of new thalamic targets.

References

1 Percheron G: The spatial organisation of information processing in the striato-pallido-nigral system; in Bignami A, Vanderhaegen JJ (eds): Basal Ganglia and Movement Disorders. Basic and Clinical Approaches. New Issues Neurosci 1991, in press.
2 Mannen H: «Noyau fermé» et «noyau ouvert». Contribution à l'étude cytoarchitectonique du tronc cérébral envisagée du point de vue du mode d'arborisation dendritique. Arch Ital Biol 1960;98:333–350.
3 Percheron G, Yelnik J, François C: Systems of coordinates for stereotactic surgery: Advantages of ventricular systems in monkeys. J Neurosci Methods 1986; 17:69–88.
4 Borke RC, Van Buren JM: The cerebello-sensory inflow to the large celled lateroventral nuclei of the chimpanzee. Anat Rec 1972;172:274.
5 Kalil K: Projections of the cerebellar and dorsal column nuclei upon the thalamus of the rhesus monkey. J Comp Neurol 1981;195:25–50.
6 Tracey DJ, Asanuma C, Jones EG, Porter R: Thalamic relay to motor cortex: afferent pathways from brain stem, cerebellum and spinal cord in monkeys. J Neurophysiol 1980;44:532–554.
7 Hirai T, Jones EG: A new parcellation of the human thalamus on the basis of histochemical staining. Brain Res Rev 1989;14:1–34.
8 Ohye C, Shibazaki T, Hirai T, Wada H, Hirato M, Kawashima Y: Further physiological observations on the ventralis intermedius neurons in the human thalamus. J Neurophysiol 1989;61:488–500.
9 Lenz FA, Tasker RR, Kwan HC, Schnider S, Kwong R, Murayama Y, Dostrowski JO, Murphy JT: Single unit analysis of the human ventral thalamic nuclear group: Correlation of thalamic 'tremor' cells with the 3–6 Hz component of Parkinsonian tremor. J Neurosci 1988;8:754–764.
10 Jones EG: Correlation and revised nomenclature of ventral nuclei in the thalamus of human and monkey. Stereotact Funct Neurosurg 1990;54/55:1–20.

11 Percheron G: The thalamic territory of cerebellar afferents in Macaques. Exp Brain Res 1975;(suppl 23):60.
12 Percheron G: The thalamic territory of cerebellar afferents and the lateral region of the thalamus of the Macaque in stereotactic ventricular coordinates. J Hirnforsch 1977;18:375–400.
13 Nauta WJH, Mehler WR: Projections of the lentiform nucleus in the monkey. Brain Res 1966;1:3–42.
14 Percheron G, François C, Parent A, Sadikot AF, Fenelon G, Yelnik J: The primate central complex as one of the basal ganglia; in Bernardi G, Carpenter MB, Di Chiara G (eds): Basal Ganglia III. New York, Plenum Press, 1991, pp 172–181.
15 Hassler R: Anatomy of the thalamus; in Schaltenbrand G, Bailey P (eds): Introduction to Stereotaxic Operations with an Atlas of the Human Brain. Stuttgart, Thieme, 1959, pp 230–290.
16 Hassler R, Mundinger F, Riechert T: Stereotaxis in Parkinson Syndrome, Berlin, Springer, 1979.
17 Jones EG: The Thalamus. New York, Plenum Press, 1985.
18 Ilinsky I, Kultas-Ilinsky K: Sagittal cytorarchitectonic maps of the *Macaca mulatta* with a revised nomenclature of the motor-related nuclei validated by observations on their connectivity. J Comp Neurol 1987;263:331–364.
19 Carpenter MB, Strominger NL: Efferent fibers of subthalamic nucleus in the monkey. A comparison of the efferent projections of the subthalamic nucleus, substantia nigra and globus pallidus. Am J Anat 1967;121:41–72.
20 Ilinsky IA, Jouandet ML, Goldman-Rakic PS: Organization of the nigrothalamocortical system in the Rhesus monkey. J Comp Neurol 1985;263:315–330.
21 Vogt C: La myéloarchitecture du thalamus du cercopithèque. J Psychol Neurol (Lpz) 1909;12:285–324.
22 Friedemann M: Die Cytoarchitektonik des Zwischenhirns der Cercopitheken mit besonderer Berücksichtigung des Thalamus opticus. J Psychol Neurol (Lpz) 1911;18:309–378.
23 Crouch RL: The nuclear configuration of the thalamus of *Macacus rhesus*. J Comp Neurol 1934;59:451–485.
24 Walker AE: A note on the thalamic nuclei of *Macaca mulatta*. J Comp Neurol 1937;66:145–155.
25 Vogt C, Vogt O: Thalamusstudien. J Psychol Neurol (Lpz) 1941;50:32–154.
26 Olszewski J: The Thalamus of the *Macaca mulatta*. Basel, Karger, 1952.
27 Van Buren JM, Borke RC: Variations and Connections of the Human Thalamus. Berlin, Springer, 1972.
28 Percheron G, François C, Yelnik J: Relations entre les ganglions de la base et le thalamus du primate. Nouvelles interprétations physiopathologiques. Rev Neurol 1986;143:337–353.
29 Jones EG, Hendry SHC: Differential calcium binding protein immunoreactivity distinguishes classes of relay neurons in monkey thalamic nuclei. Eur J Neurosci 1989;1:222–246.

G. Percheron, MD, INSERM Unité 106, Pavillon Claude-Bernard, Hôpital de la Salpêtrière, 47, Bd de l'Hôpital, F–75651 Paris Cedex 13 (France)

Proceedings of the 2nd International Workshop on Microphysiological Recordings during Stereotactic Neurosurgery: Motor Thalamus, October 1–2, 1989, Nikko, Japan
Stereotact Funct Neurosurg 1993;60:42–61

Cortical Connections of the Motor Thalamic Nuclei in the Japanese Monkey, *Macaca fuscata*

K. Nakano[a], *Y. Hasegawa*[b], *T. Kayahara*[a], *A. Tokushige*[b], *Y. Kuga*[a]

[a] Department of Anatomy, School of Medicine, Mie University, Mie; [b] Department of Anatomy, Faculty of Medicine, Kagoshima University, Kagoshima, Japan

Key Words. Thalamus · Basal ganglia · Motor cortex · Premotor cortex · Supplementary motor cortex · Monkey

Abstract. Our findings revealed the nucleus ventralis lateralis pars oralis (VLo) projection to motor area, and the nucleus ventralis anterior pars principalis (VApc) projections to the premotor and supplementary motor areas (SMA). The VLo gave rise to thalamocortical projections terminating in the superficial half of layer I, mainly in the forelimb motor area. The VApc gave rise to the superficial projections to the post-arcuate premotor area around the arcuate genu and arcuate spur as well as SMA. We suggested that the medial pallidal segment projects to the motor area via VLo, and to the premotor area and SMA via VApc. We also proposed that the premotor area and SMA receive cerebellar afferents via nucleus ventralis lateralis pars caudalis and area X.

Introduction

The application of modern axonal transport techniques has shed new light upon the organization of thalamocortical connections. These studies have been reviewed briefly by Jones [9]. Since Shell and Strick's [23] description, the nucleus ventralis lateralis pars oralis (VLo) projection to the supplementary motor area (SMA) has been accepted by many researchers. Recently, Jones [10] divided the ventral thalamic nuclei into four channels relaying pallidal, substantia nigral, cerebellar,

1011–6125/93/0603–0042 $ 2.75/0

and lemniscal information separately to the cerebral cortex. He attempted to divide the ventral motor thalamic nuclei simply into the anterior and posterior portions, relaying pallidal and cerebellar afferents to the premotor and motor cortices, respectively.

However, a number of uncertainties continue to exist regarding the cortical projection from the motor thalamic nuclei. The thalamic integration of diverse information from spinal cord, cerebellum, and basal ganglia was suggested by Darian-Smith et al. [4]. The VLo projection to the motor cortex has been reported by a number of authors [4–6, 12, 13, 15–17, 25]. This is not in complete agreement with evidence that the cerebello-thalamo-cortical pathway projects exclusively to area 4 [11, 26]. The nucleus ventralis posterolateralis pars oralis (VPLo) projections to SMA and postarcuate cortex were reported by Darian-Smith et al. [4]. In the present study axonal transport techniques by horseradish peroxidase (HRP) and tritiated amino acid were used to clarify the cortical projections from the individual motor thalamic nuclei. Preliminary reports of some of these data have been presented earlier in abstract form [18, 19].

Material and Methods

The experiments were carried out on 54 macaque monkeys *(Macaca fuscata)* of either sex with weights ranging from 2.8 to 12 kg. Each monkey was anesthetized with ketamine hydrochloride (Ketalar, 10 mg/kg) and sodium pentobarbital (15–30 mg/kg), and placed in a David Kopf stereotaxic head holder. Then a tracer was injected into the cortical area or stereotactically into the motor thalamic nuclei.

WGA-HRP Tracing Experiments

Single or multiple injections of 2% wheat germ agglutinin-conjugated horseradish peroxidase (WGA-HRP) were placed ipsilaterally or bilaterally in the various portions of the frontal lobe, 1–1.5 mm below cortical surface, by manual pressure (0.1–0.3 μl), using a glass micropipette attached to a Hamilton syringe.

After a survival time of 24–48 h, the monkeys were deeply reanesthetized with ketamine, and perfused through the left cardiac ventricle with 500 ml of 0.9% saline followed by 3,000 ml of freshly prepared fixative (1.25% glutaraldehyde-0.1% paraformaldehyde mixture in a 0.1 *M* phosphate buffer, pH 7.4), and finally by 1,000 ml of the same buffer containing 10% sucrose. The brains were removed, placed in 30% sucrose in the same buffer at 4 °C, and cut serially into 50 μm thick sections on a freezing microtome. The sections were processed by diaminobenzidine (DAB) or tetramethyl benzidine (TMB) for HRP histochemistry.

Autoradiographic Tracing Experiments

The ^{3}H-leucine was evaporated under nitrogen gas, and then reconstituted in concentration of 20–100 μCi/μl with sterile saline. Also, ^{3}H-leucine was injected into the various parts of the frontal lobe (3–5 μl), or stereotactically into the motor thalamic nuclei (0.3–0.5 μl). After 5–9 days of survival, the monkeys were perfused with 10% buffered neutral formalin again under deep anesthesia. Following postfixing of the brains in the same fixative, autoradiography was performed on 7-μm thick sections cut on paraffin microtome and mounted on slides. Slides were dipped in Sakura NRM2 emulsion, exposed at 4 °C for 4–20 weeks, developed, and then counterstained with cresyl violet.

Retrogradely labeled neurons or anterogradely labeled terminals and fibers were observed under bright- and darkfield illumination. The nomenclature of the thalamic nuclei was adapted from Olszewski [27].

Results

The following description consists of two parts: (1) data obtained from our WGA-HRP studies on the thalamocortical connections, and (2) autoradiographic studies on the thalamocortical and corticothalamic connections.

WGA-HRP Studies

WGA-HRP injections were made in 9 cases in the various portions of the dorso-rostral part of the premotor cortex (6DR) (fig. 1), the region between the midline and superior arcuate sulcus (As). In these cases labeled neurons in the motor thalamus were observed in the nucleus ventralis anterior pars principalis (VApc), nucleus ventralis lateralis pars caudalis (VLc), area X, nucleus ventralis lateralis pars medialis (VLm), and nucleus ventralis lateralis pars postrema (VLps). Distribution of labeled neurons in these nuclei was shown in detail in a single case (M 476L) in figure 2A. The injection in this case was made at the center of 6DR. Labeled neurons in VApc were located along the lateral portion of the rostral VApc, and caudally these labeled neurons were concentrated in the dorsal part of VApc. Labeled neurons in VLc were observed in its dorsomedial portion. Labeled neurons in area X and VLps distributed in the medial half of these nuclei. There were also a few labeled neurons in the dorsal portion of nucleus parafascicularis (Pf) (fig. 2A).

When the injection was made in the rostral part of 6DR, labeled neurons in the VApc, area X, and VLc were shifted more medially.

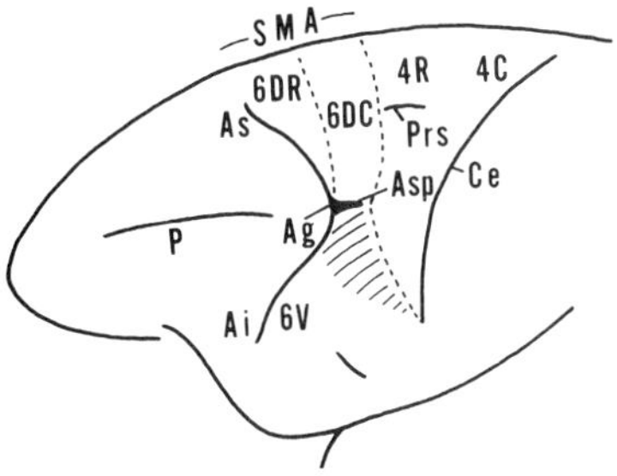

Fig. 1. Subdivisions of the premotor and motor cortex. SMA = Supplementary motor area; 6DR = dorsorostral part of area 6; 6DC = dorsocaudal part of area 6; 4R = rostral part of area 4; 4C = caudal part of area 4; 6V = ventral part of area 6; As = superior branch of arcuate sulcus; Ai = inferior branch of arcuate sulcus; Ag = arcuate genu; Asp = arcuate spur; Ce = central sulcus; P = principal sulcus; Prs = superior precentral sulcus.

When the injection was made in the transitional region between 6DR and area 9, labeled neurons were seen in the lateral part of VAmc, and in the medial parts of VApc, VLc and area X. In a case in which three injections were made in the ventral 6DR close to the superior arcuate sulcus, the labeled neurons were located in the dorsomedial portions of VApc, VLc and VAmc, and in the medial portion of area X. Similar distribution of labeled neurons were observed following an injection in the corner between the superior arcuate sulcus (As) and arcuate spur (Asp).

WGA-HRP injections were made in the dorsocaudal portion of the premotor cortex (6DC) (fig. 1), corresponding to a premotor region between the midline and arcuate spur (Asp), caudal to the 6DR and rostral to the superior precentral sulcal area (4R), in 8 cases. With WGA-HRP injection in the 6DC, rostral to the superior precentral sulcus, labeled neurons in the motor thalamus were found in the VApc, VLc, area X, VLm and VLps (fig. 2B). Labeled neurons in VApc were seen in the lateral portion of VApc, medial to the nucleus ventralis lateralis pars oralis (VLo). Some labeled neurons were scattered in the transitional zone between VApc and VLo. Labeled neurons in VLc and area X were seen in the intermediate zone of the mediolateral extent of these nuclei. The arrangement of labeled neurons in VLc was parallel to the dorsomedial margin of VLc. Labeled neurons were present also

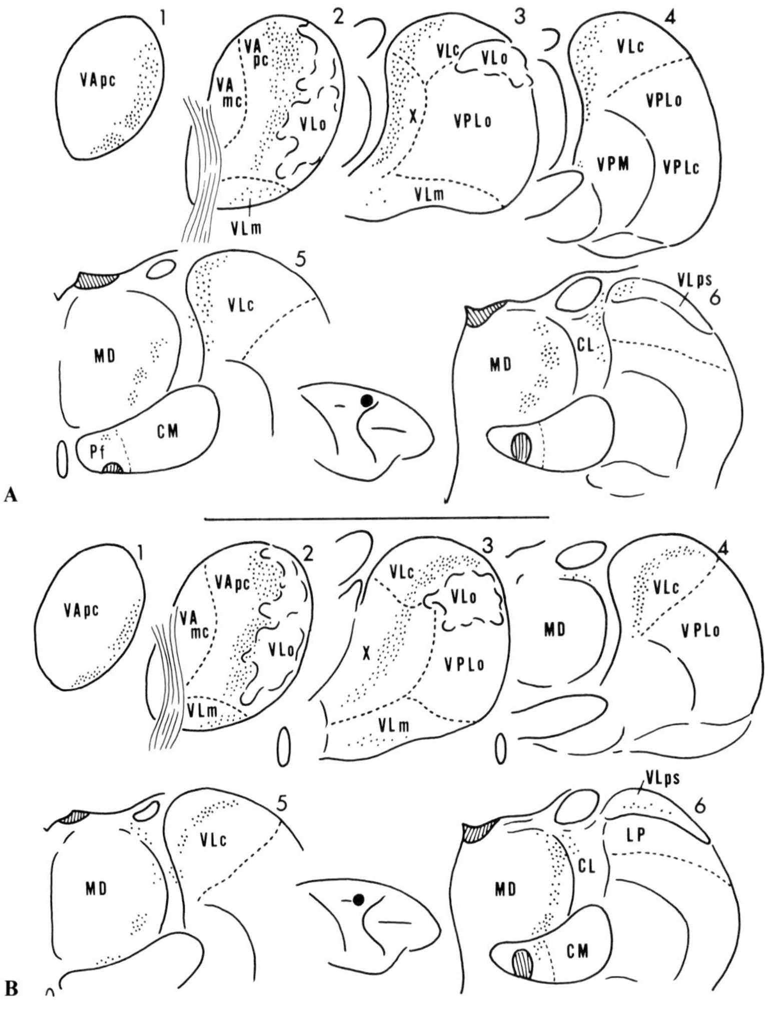

Fig. 2. Distribution of retrograde labeled thalamic neurons following WGA-HRP injection in the dorsorostral part of area 6 (6DR) (M 476L) (**A**), dorsocaudal part of area 6 (6DC) (M 454) (**B**), and the ventral part of area 6 (6V) (M 476R) (**C**). Numbers indicate rostrocaudal sequence. Each dot represents one labeled thalamic neuron. Injection sites (black areas) were indicated in the middle lower part in **A** and **B** and in the lower right corner in **C**. CM = Nucleus centrum medianum; CL = nucleus centralis lateralis. Other labels of thalamic nuclei are those of Olszewski [27].

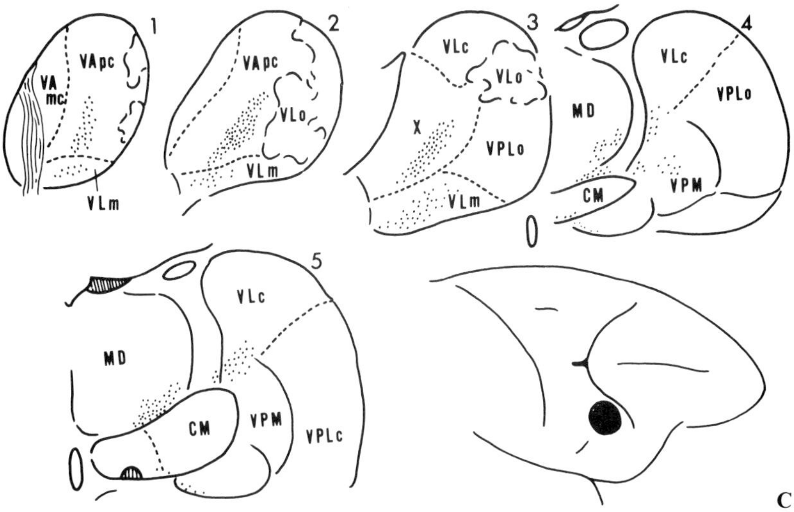

C

in the lateral part of the caudal half of the nucleus medialis dorsalis (MD) and less densely in the dorsolateral part of Pf (fig. 2B). A small number of labeled neurons was detected in the ventromedial portion of VPLo in some sections. In a case in which the injection site in 6DC was located more rostrodorsally, labeled neurons in the motor thalamus were distributed somewhat more medially than those in the above cases.

WGA-HRP injections were made in the region ventrocaudal to the arcuate genu (Ag) and ventral to the arcuate spur (Asp) (diagonal shaded area in fig. 1) in three cases. In these cases, labeled neurons in the motor thalamus were found in the VApc, VLo, VLc, VLm, area X and VPLo. The labeled neurons were also located in the transitional zone between VApc and VLo, as well as in the transitional zones of the caudal VLo-VLc, VPLo-area X, and of the VLc-VPLo.

WGA-HRP injections were made in the ventral part of the premotor cortex (6V in fig. 1) in 8 cases. In a representative case (M 476R) in which the injection site involved a large region ventral to the rostral half of the inferior arcuate sulcus (Ai), labeled neurons were found in the ventral parts of VApc, and area X, the medial half of VLm and the ventrolateral MD (fig. 2C).

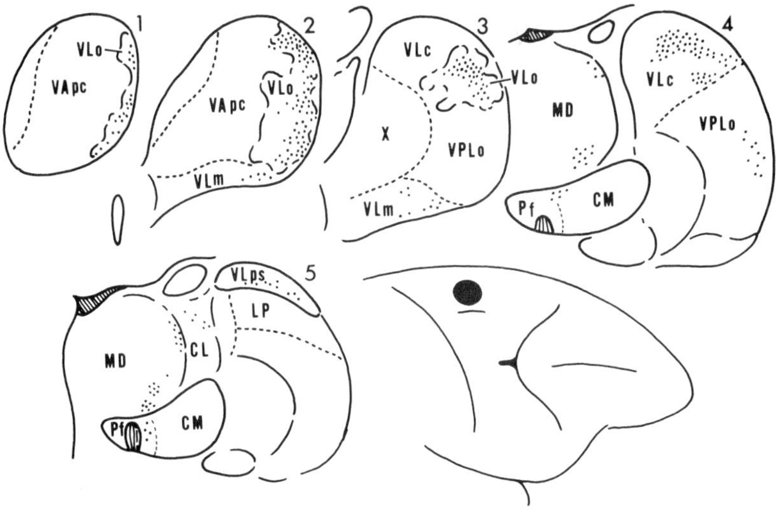

Fig. 3. Distribution of retrograde labeled thalamic neurons following WGA-HRP injection in a region medial to the superior precentral sulcus (M 441). The injection site (black area) is indicated in the lower right part of the figure. See figure 2 for details.

WGA-HRP injections were made in the various parts of the motor cortex in 26 cases. With an injection in the region medial to the superior precentral sulcus (M 441), labeled neurons were seen in the VLo, VLm, VLc, VLps and in the transitional zone between the nucleus centrum medianum (CM) and Pf (fig. 3). No labeled neurons were observed in VPLo, except for a few labeled neurons in the ventrocaudal part of this nucleus, whereas, with an injection caudal to that of M 441, labeled neurons were observed in VPLo in addition to VLo, VLm, VLc, VLps and CM. In this case, labeled neurons were located in the lateral portions of VLo and VPLo (but not in the lateral margin), and in the ventrolateral part of VLc. Labeled neurons were detected in the dorsomedial portion of CM. After an injection in the region caudal to the superior precentral sulcus, labeled neurons were found also in both the VLo and VPLo.

Following injections in the dorsomedial part of the motor cortex (hindlimb representation), labeled neurons were noted in the lateral parts of VLo, VLm, and VPLo, and in the ventrolateral parts of VLc and MD (fig. 4A, 5A, 8A). Labeled neurons in CM were localized in its dorsomedial part. With injections in the ventrolateral part of the motor

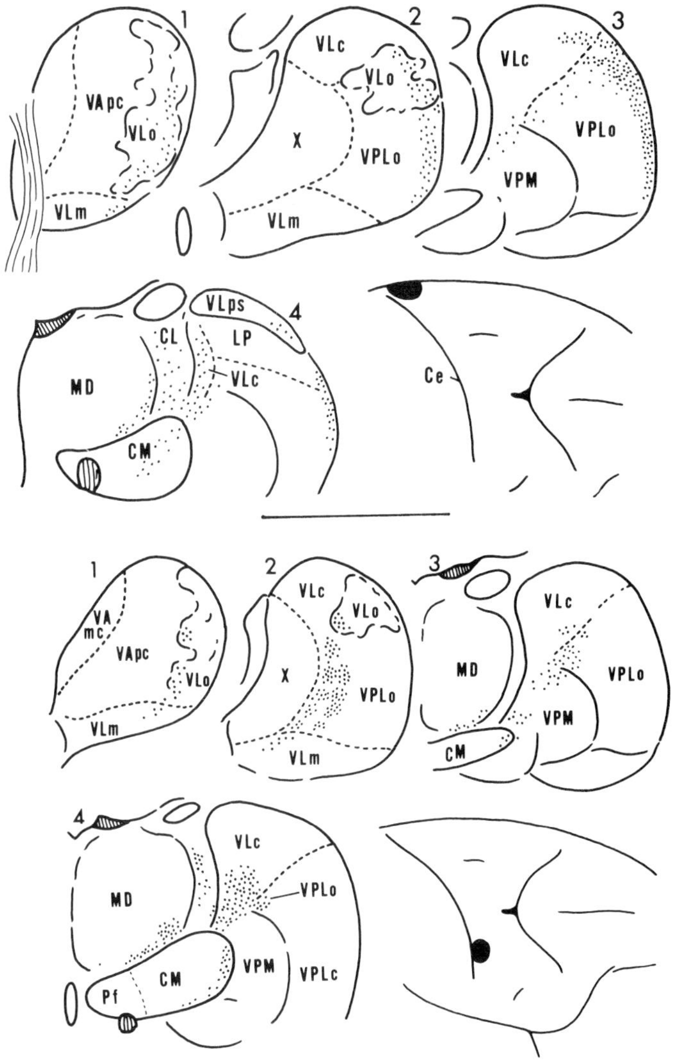

A

B

Fig. 4. Distribution of retrograde labeled thalamic neurons following WGA-HRP injection in **(A)** the dorsomedial part of area 4 (hindlimb representation) (M 235); **(B)** ventral part (face representation) (M 242), and **(C)** the intermediate part of area 4 (forelimb representation) (M 195). The injection sites were indicated in the lower right parts of **A–C**. See figure 2 for details.

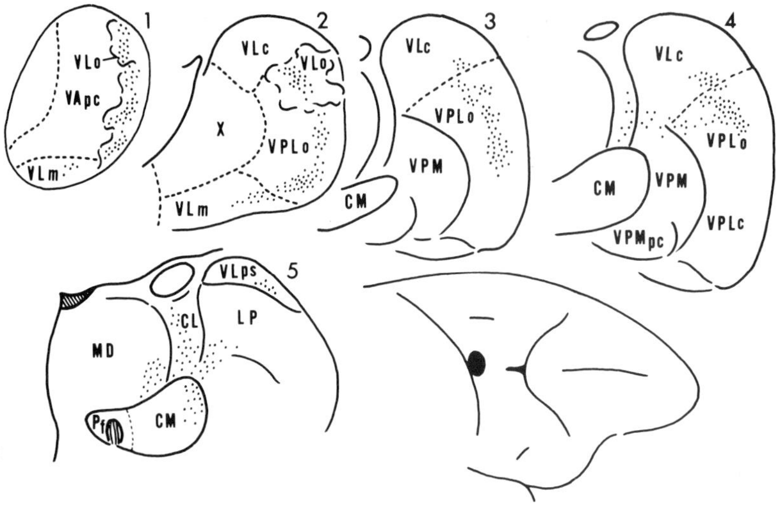

4C

cortex (face representation by Sessle and Wiesendanger [24]), labeled neurons were seen in the medial parts of VLo and VPLo. Labeled neurons in CM were located in its ventrolateral part (fig. 4B, 8A). In these cases no labeled neurons were detected in the most rostral part of VLo. With WGA-HRP injections in the intermediate part of the motor area (forelimb representation by Sessle and Wiesendanger [24]), labeled neurons in the VLo, VPLo, VLc and CM were distributed in the intermediate zone between the territories projecting to the hindlimb and face motor areas with some overlap (fig. 4C, 8A). Labeled neurons in VLo and VLc were more dense after WGA-HRP injections in the rostral part of the motor cortex (4R in fig. 1), than those in the more caudal part of the motor cortex (4C in fig. 1). VLc neurons projecting to the motor cortex were predominantly encountered in its ventrocaudal portion (fig. 3, 4). No labeled neurons were detected in the rostral VLc following motor cortex injections.

In 14 cases, WGA-HRP was injected in the various portions of the SMA and its adjacent areas. An injection in the central portion of SMA resulted in labeling of neurons in the VApc, VLc, VLm, area X and in the transitional zone between the Pf and CM as well as in the lateral MD and nucleus centralis lateralis (CL) (fig. 6). Labeled neurons in VApc were located in its lateral part at the level of rostral

A 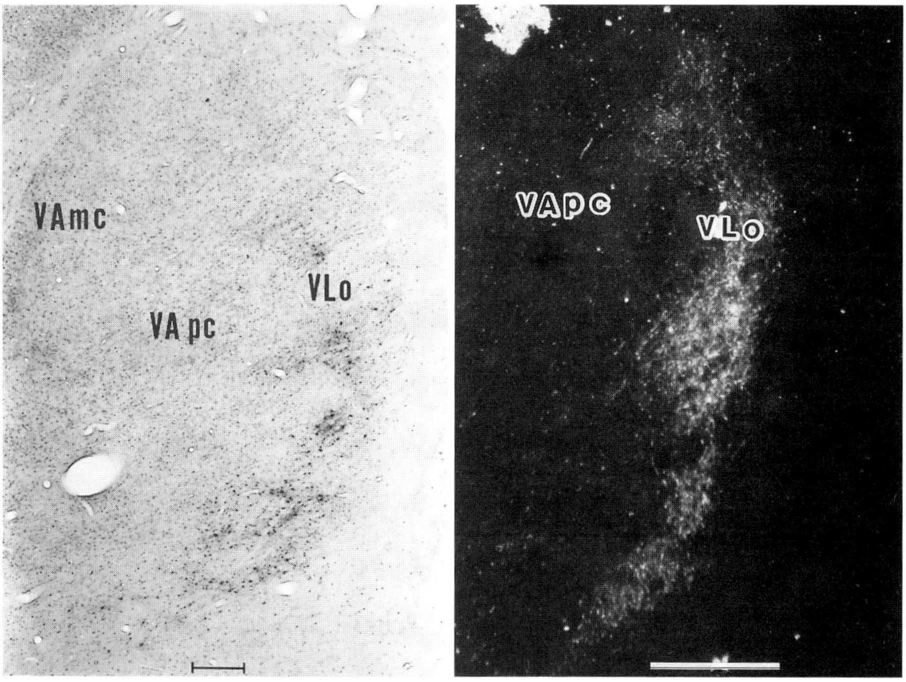 B

Fig. 5. **A** Photomicrograph of a coronal section of the thalamus showing labeled neurons in VLo following WGA-HRP injection in the dorsomedial part of rostral motor cortex (M 440). **B** Dark-field photomicrograph of a coronal section of the thalamus showing anterograde labeled terminals in VLo following tritiated leucine injection in the dorsomedial part of rostral motor cortex (M 120). Bar = 500 μm.

VApc, and caudally located in the lateral two-thirds of the nucleus, but not in VLo (fig. 7A). Labeled neurons in area X were noted in its lateral part. Followed caudally, labeled neurons in the VLc were confined in the ventrolateral to ventral portions of the nucleus. There were also only a few labeled neurons in the VLps (fig. 6). These labeled neurons of the motor thalamus shifted more medially with injections in the rostral portion of SMA. Labeled neurons were observed in the transitional zone between VApc and VLo, after injections in the caudal portion of SMA. Following injections in the rostral portion (4R in fig. 1) of the medial motor cortex, labeled neurons were detected in VLo, but not in VApc.

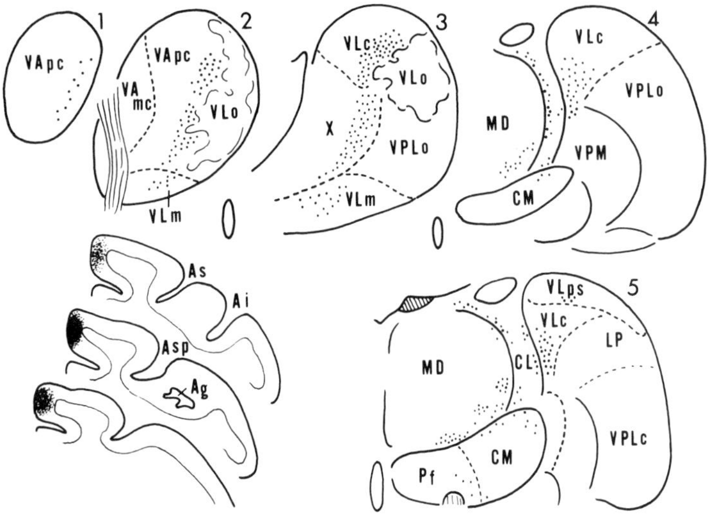

Fig. 6. Distribution of retrograde labeled thalamic neurons following WGA-HRP injection in the supplementary motor area (SMA) (M 448). The injection site (black area) is indicated in the lower left part of the figure. As = superior branch of arcuate sulcus; Ai = inferior branch of arcuate sulcus; Ag = arcuate genu; Asp = arcuate spur. See figure 2 for details.

^{3}H-Leucine Injections in the Frontal Cortex

As the thalamic nuclei connect reciprocally with the cerebral cortex, ^{3}H-leucine was placed in the various portions of premotor and motor areas as well as SMA in 24 cases. Following ^{3}H-leucine injection in the central part of SMA, anterogradely labeled terminals were observed in similar regions, where retrogradely labeled neurons of HRP were seen with the WGA-HRP injection made in the central SMA. Terminal labeling was observed in the lateral part of VApc (fig. 7B), and also in the lateral half of area X. Terminal labeling was dense in VApc, but none was found in VLo (fig. 7B). Terminal labeling in VLc was mainly manifest in its ventrolateral portion, and displaced caudally in the intermediate to ventromedial portions. There were also labeled terminals in the ventrolateral part of caudal MD and in the transitional zone between CM and Pf.

With ^{3}H-leucine injections in the distinct portions of the premotor cortex, terminal labeling was located in each thalamic territory project-

A 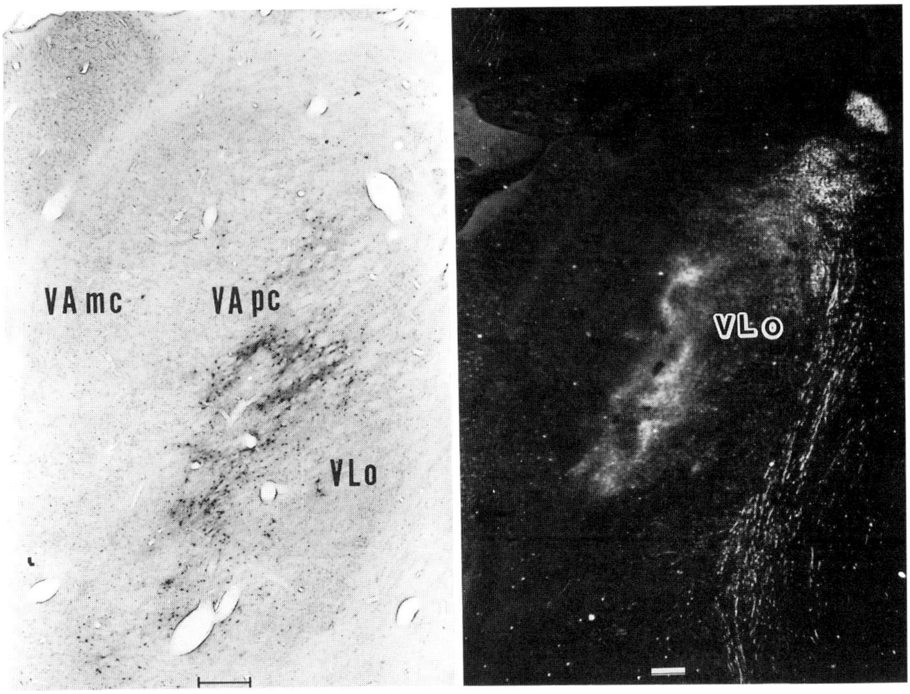 B

Fig. 7. **A** Photomicrograph of a coronal section of the thalamus showing labeled neurons in the lateral VApc following WGA-HRP injection in the supplementary motor area (SMA) (M 448). **B** Dark-field photomicrograph of a coronal section of the thalamus showing anterograde labeled terminals in the lateral VApc following tritiated leucine injection in the SMA (M 111). Bar = 500 μm.

ing to these cortical portions. Following ^{3}H-leucine injection in the rostral 6DR and adjacent area 9, dense terminal labeling could be seen in the lateral VAmc and medial VApc, and in the medial zones of area X and VLC. With injection in 6DC, dense terminal labeling resulted in the dorsal to medial parts of VApc, and in the medial parts (except for the medial margin) of VLc and area X. After injection in the ventral part of the premotor area (6V in fig. 1), ventral to the inferior arcuate sulcus, terminal labeling was observed in the ventromedial part of VApc, and in the dorsomedial part of VLm. No terminal labeling was seen in VLo and VLc. Only fibers of passage were labeled in VLo.

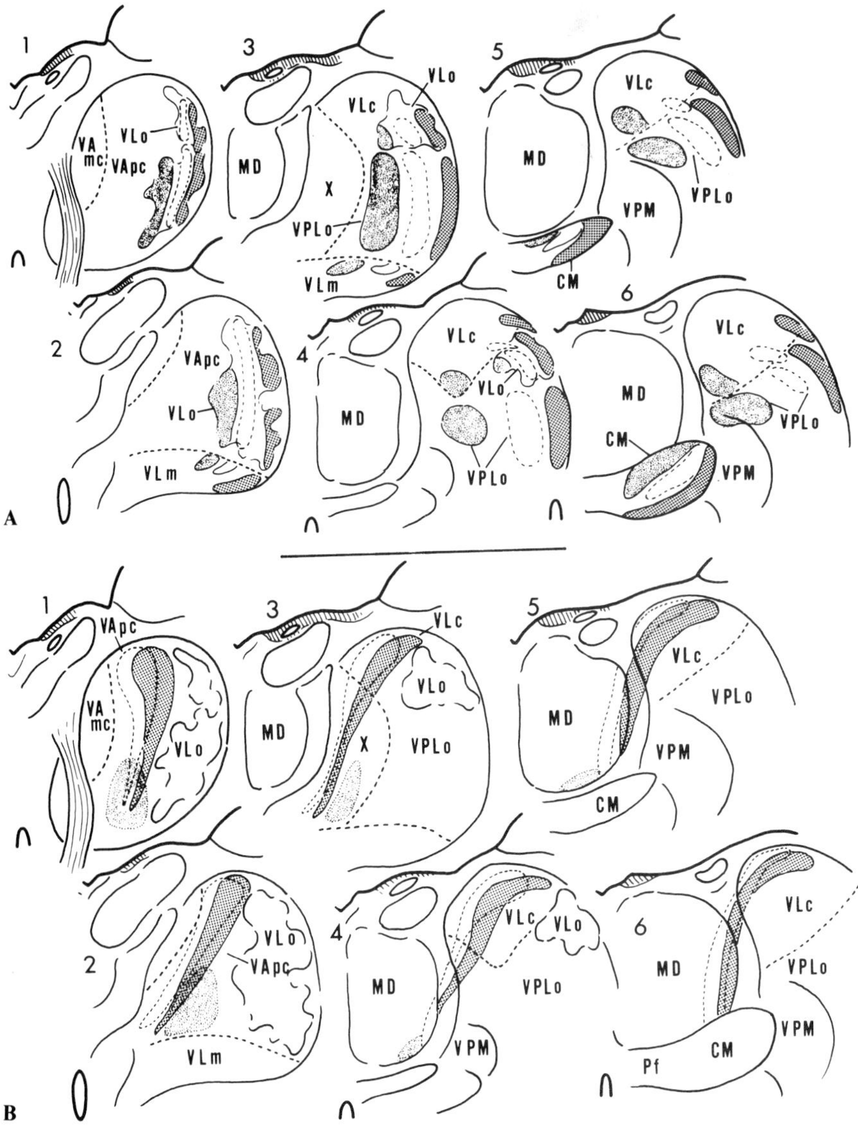

Fig. 8. Semidiagrammatic outlines of (**A**) the territories of motor thalamic nuclei connecting with motor area (dotted area = hindlimb territory; area surrounded by dotted line = forelimb territory; shaded area = face territory), and (**B**) connecting with premotor area (dotted area = 6DC territory, area surrounded by dotted line = 6DR territory, shaded area = 6V territory). See figure 2 for details.

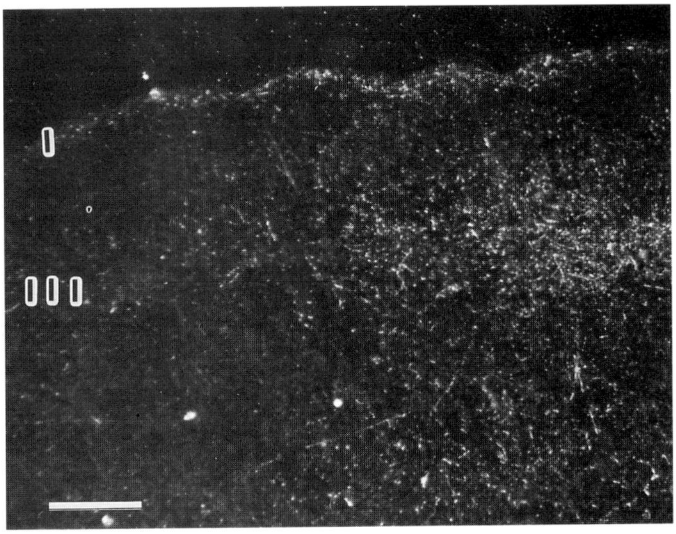

Fig. 9. Dark-field photomicrograph showing terminal labeling in the superficial (superficial half of lamina I) and deep (lamina III) layers of the rostral motor cortex around the superior precentral sulcus following tritiated leucine injection in VLo (M 25). Bar = 300 μm.

^{3}H-leucine was placed in the various portions of the motor area in 11 cases, in which terminal labeling was found also in the thalamic territories presumably projecting to the injection site. The mediolateral topography was also observed as seen in the HRP findings. A slab of terminal labeling was seen in the VLo (fig. 5B), VLc, VLm, and VPLo. This slab is not always present beyond nuclear boundaries, but is interrupted with each cytoarchitectonic boundaries as indicated in figure 8A.

^{3}H-Leucine Injections in Motor Thalamus

^{3}H-Leucine was injected in the motor thalamic nuclei in 13 cases. With ^{3}H-leucine injection in the ventral part of VAmc, terminal labeling was seen in the superficial layer (lamina I) and deep layers (lamina III-V) of the banks of the arcuate genu (Ag in fig. 1) and arcuate spur (Asp in fig. 1) as well as in the deep layers of the banks of the superior and inferior arcuate sulci, and in the layers of the prefrontal cortex adjacent to these sulci (areas 8 and 9). Following injections in VApc, terminal labeling was observed in the superficial layer and deep layers around the arcuate genu and spur, and in the 6DC and SMA. Terminal labeling only in the deep layers was found in the ventral part of area 6 (6V in fig. 1) and ventral bank of the cingulate sulcus. With injections in VLo, superficial terminal labeling was found in the ventrolateral half of motor area (face and forelimb representations). The terminal labeling in the superficial and deep layers was also evident in the rostral motor area (fig. 9).

With a VLm injection, the terminal labeling in the superficial cortical layer was seen in the arcuate spur and anterior bank of the central sulcus of forelimb and face motor areas. Only deep cortical termination was observed following VLc, VPLo or area X injection. With area X injections, deep cortical termination was detected in the arcuate premotor area and banks of the arcuate sulcus. Following VLc injections, deep cortical termination was present in the 6DC and rostral motor area (4R in fig. 1), around the superior precentral sulcus, as well as SMA. Injections in VPLo resulted in deep cortical termination in the caudal motor area (4C in fig. 1) as well as in the fundus of the central sulcus (area 3a). These autoradiographic studies on the thalamocortical projections will be described in detail elsewhere.

Discussion

On the basis of our findings, the approximate thalamic territories connecting with the subdivisions of premotor and motor areas are shown diagrammatically in figure 8. The thalamic territory of 6DR (area surround by dotted line in fig. 8B) is located more medially than that of 6DC (dotted area) with some mediolateral overlap. The thalamic territory connecting with each face, forelimb and hindlimb representation of motor area occupies the medial, intermediate and lateral bands, respectively, with mediolateral topography in VLc, VLo and VPLo. The thalamic territory connecting with the motor area occupies the ventrocaudal part of VLc.

Our findings indicated the VLo projection to the motor area. The rostral portion of the motor cortex, which is confined to the region around the superior precentral sulcus, receives afferent inputs from VLo, but not from VPLo. The VLo has been considered to be the relay nucleus of the pallidal projection to the premotor area [2, 9]. Schell and Strick [23] reported the VLo projection to SMA, and this finding was supported by some authors [6, 28]. Darian-Smith et al. [4] also reported the VLo projection to SMA, but in their case the neurons projecting to SMA were mainly located in the ventrolateral part of VLc, with only a few neurons in VLo.

In the cases under study here, HRP injections made in the center of SMA produced labeled neurons mainly in VApc, but not in VLo (fig. 7A). Injections in the rostral SMA resulted in labeled neurons in the more medial region of VApc. There is a difference in the mediolateral distribution of labeled neurons in VApc, depending on the injection site. The rostral SMA receives afferent inputs from the more medial VApc. The VLo projection to caudal SMA was indicated by Wiesendanger and Wiesendanger [28]. Although the possibility of VLo projection to the caudal SMA was not denied, quite intensely labeled neurons in VLo were found following injection in the rostral motor area. We considered that the transitional area between the VApc and VLo projects to the caudal SMA. The cytoarchitectonic identification of the SMA and VLo is critical. The caudal boundaries of SMA are identifiable from the motor area on the basis of the Betz cells in the latter. The VLo is well demarcated on cytoarchitectonic grounds. Neurons in this nucleus are well stained and dense.

As VLo and VApc receives afferent inputs from the medial pallidal segment (GPm) [14], the premotor and rostral motor areas appear to receive GPm afferents via VApc and VLo, respectively. Our data strongly suggested that the motor cortex is controlled by the basal ganglia in addition to the cerebellar nuclei. Neurons in VPLo were more strongly labeled after HRP injections located in the more caudal motor area. The basal ganglia presumably affect the rostral motor area, whereas the cerebellar nuclei affect the caudal motor area. The VPLo projection to the caudal motor area was also described by Jones et al. [11].

Our autoradiographic findings indicated a deep thalamocortical (T-C) projection from the VPLo to the motor area, whereas there were superficial (lamina I) and deep thalamocortical projections from the VApc and VLo to the premotor and motor areas. The superficial T-C projections were observed mainly in the regions caudal to the arcuate genu, and forelimb motor area. These areas seem to receive GPm information via VApc and VLo. The cortical areas are also heavily connected with SMA [19]. The functional significance of the superficial T-C projection, which seems to transport GPm information to the forelimb motor area and the arcuate genu area, is interesting for its control of complex motor function. The superficial T-C responses, however, were recorded in the monkey motor cortex following cerebellar nuclear stimulation [22]. The pallidal projection to motor area via VLo was recorded by the stimulating method [21]. According to Jinnai et al. [8], neurons receiving pallidal inhibition project to the lamina I of the sigmoid gyrus, while neurons receiving cerebellar excitation do so to the deeper layers in the cat.

Our data indicated the VApc and area X projections to the premotor area and SMA. As area X and VLc receives cerebellar afferents [2], it is considered that the cerebellar nuclei also project to the premotor area and SMA via area X and VLc in addition to motor area projection through VPLo. Our findings suggest that the motor and premotor areas receive both afferent inputs from the pallidal and cerebellar nuclei through the motor thalamus. Ilinsky and Kultas-Ilinsky [7] also reported the possibility that both GPm and cerebellum control thalamic output to the premotor as well as the motor cortices. However, each thalamocortical pathway to the premotor, SMA and motor areas is considered to be associated with a distinct subcortical input [2, 10, 23]. Schell and Strick [23] considered that direct interactions between the three systems are largely limited to the cortical level, where the SMA, arcuate premotor, and motor areas are reciprocally interconnected with one another. On the other hand, the thalamic integration of diverse information from spinal cord, cerebellum, and basal ganglia was suggested by Darian-Smith et al. [4]. Matelli et al. [16] suggested that the ventral area 6 (their area F5) and caudal area 4 are under cerebellar influence via area X and VPLo, and control distal movements. They also suggested that pallidal information is transported to rostral area 4 and a region (their area F4) between area 4 and area F5 via VLo, and control proximal movements.

Although we suggested dual control of the basal ganglia and cerebellum on the premotor and motor areas, the basal ganglia and cerebellar channel through the motor thalamus are considered to process by different mechanisms, as suggested by Jones [10] and Alexander et al. [1].

On the basis of the present autoradiographic and HRP studies, VLc projects to the rostral motor area, around the superior precentral sulcus, and to the 6DC premotor area. The VLc projection to the ventral premotor area was not observed in our cases. No superficial T-C

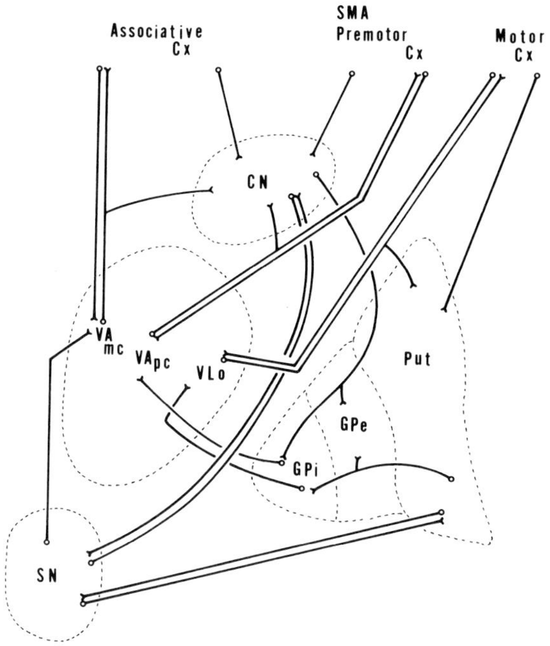

Fig. 10. Summary diagram showing VAmc, VApc, and VLo connections with frontal lobe and basal ganglia on the basis of our data.

projection from VLc was detected in this autoradiographic study. The VLc appears to project to the deeper layers of the dorsomedial part of the 6DC and the rostral motor area. The VLc projection to the rostral motor area was reported also by Jones et al. [11]. Our data also indicated the nucleus ventralis anterior pars magnocellularis (VAmc) projections to the prefrontal cortex, especially to the frontal eye field (area 8), the banks of the caudal part of the principal sulcus, and the arcuate sulcal area. The substantia nigra influences the prefrontal cortex and SMA via VAmc [6]. As VAmc is a nigral territory of the motor thalamus [3, 6], our present findings also corroborate support the nigral influence on the prefrontal cortex.

The VLo projects also to the putamen, which is the main destination of the corticostriatal projection from the motor cortex; the VApc projects to the lateral part of the caudate nucleus (CN) and rostral putamen, which are the destination of the premotor cortical afferents, and the VAmc to the medial CN, which is the territory of the frontal association cortex [20]. It seems likely that these thalamostriatal fibers may represent collaterals of thalamocortical projections as well as the striatal projections from the intralaminar thalamic nuclei. The neostriatum is functionally and anatomically heterogeneous, and it is proposed that the cortico-striato-thalamocortical circuits are segregated and organized in a parallel manner [1]. On the basis of our present and previous studies [3, 14, 18–20], we summarized the motor thalamic connections as indicated in figure 10.

Acknowledgements

This study was partly supported by grants for scientific research (Nos. 557017, 56570022, and 57570023) from the Ministry of Education of the Japanese Government.

References

1 Alexander GE, DeLong MR, Strick PL: Parallel organization of functionally integrated circuits linking basal ganglia and cortex. Annu Rev Neurosci 1986;9:357–382.
2 Asanuma C, Thach WT, Jones EG: Distribution of cerebellar terminations and their relation to other afferent terminations in the ventral lateral thalamic region of the monkey. Brain Res Rev 1983;5:237–265.
3 Carpenter MB, Nakano K, Kim R: Nigrothalamic projections in the monkey demonstrated by autoradiographic technics. J Comp Neurol 1976;165:401–415.
4 Darian-Smith C, Darian-Smith I, Cheema SS: Thalamic projections to sensorimotor cortex in the macaque monkey: Use of multiple retrograde fluorescent tracers. J Comp Neurol 1990;299:17–46.
5 Ghosh S, Brinkman C, Porter R: A quantitative study of the distribution of neurons projecting to the precentral motor cortex in the monkey *(M. fascicularis)*. J Comp Neurol 1987;259:424–444.
6 Ilinsky IA, Jouandet ML, Goldman-Rakic PS: Organization of the nigrothalamocortical system in the rhesus monkey. J Comp Neurol 1985;236:315–330.
7 Ilinsky IA, Kultas-Ilinsky K: Sagittal cytoarchitectonic maps of the macaca mulatta thalamus with a revised nomenclature of the motor-related nuclei validated by observations on their connectivity. J Comp Neurol 1987;262:331–364.
8 Jinnai K, Nambu A, Yoshida S: Thalamic afferents to layer I of anterior sigmoid cortex originating from the VA-VL neurons with entopeduncular input. Exp Brain Res 1987;69:67–76.
9 Jones EG: The Thalamus. New York, Plenum Press, 1985.
10 Jones EG: Correlation and revised nomenclature of ventral nuclei in the thalamus of human and monkey. Stereotact Funct Neurosurg 1989;54/55:1–20.
11 Jones EG, Wise SP, Coulter JD: Differential thalamic relationship of sensory motor and parietal cortical fields in monkeys. J Comp Neurol 1979;183:833–882.

12 Kalil K: Neuroanatomical organization of the primate motor system; in Otto OA (ed): Multidisciplinary Perspectives in Event-Related Brain Potential Research. Washington, Environmental Protection Agency, 1978, pp 112–123.
13 Kievit J, Kuypers HGJM: Organization of the thalamocortical connexions to the frontal lobe in the rhesus monkey. Exp Brain Res 1977;29:299–322.
14 Kim R, Nakano K, Jayaraman A, Carpenter MB: Projections of the globus pallidus and adjacent structures. An autoradiographic study in the monkey. J Comp Neurol 1976;169:263–290.
15 Leichnetz GR: Afferent and efferent connections of the dorsolateral precentral gyrus (area 4, hand/arm region) in the macaque monkey, with comparisons to area 8. J Comp Neurol 1986;254:460–492.
16 Matelli M, Luppino G, Fogassi L, Rizzolatti G: Thalamic input to inferior area 6 and area 4 in the macaque monkey. J Comp Neurol 1989;280:468–488.
17 Miyata M, Sasaki K: HRP studies on thalamocortical neurons related to the cerebellocerebral projection in the monkey. Brain Res 1983;274:213–224.
18 Nakano K, Kohno M, Hasegawa Y, Tokushige A, Sasaki K: Anatomical study of superficial and deep thalamocortical projections in the monkey. Neurosci Lett 1984;(suppl 17):S64.
19 Nakano K, Kohno M, Hasegawa Y, Tokushige A: The neuron distribution projecting to the supplementary motor area and adjacent area in the monkey. Neurosci Res 1985;(suppl 1):S78.
20 Nakano K, Hasegawa Y, Tokushige A, Nakagawa S, Kayahara T, Mizuno N: Topographical projections from the thalamus, subthalamic nucleus and pedunculopontine tegmental nucleus to the striatum in the Japanese monkey, *Macaca fuscata*. Brain Res 1990;537:54–68.
21 Nambu A, Yoshida S, Jinnai K: Projection on the motor cortex of thalamic neurons with pallidal input in the monkey. Exp Brain Res 1988;71:658–662.
22 Sasaki K, Kawaguchi S, Oka H, Sakai M, Mizuno N: Electrophysiological studies on the cerebello-cerebral projections in monkeys. Exp Brain Res 1976;24:495–507.
23 Schell GR, Strick PL: The origin of thalamic inputs to the arcuate premotor and supplementary motor areas. J Neurosci 1984;4:539–560.
24 Sessle BJ, Wiesendanger M: Structural and functional definition of the motor cortex in the monkey *(Macaca fascicularis)*. J Physiol 1982;323:245–265.
25 Strick PL: Anatomical analysis of ventrolateral thalamic input to primate motor cortex. J Neurophysiol 1976;39:1020–1031.
26 Tracey DJ, Asanuma C, Jones EG, Porter R: Thalamic relay to motor cortex: Afferent pathways from brainstem, cerebellum, and spinal cord in monkeys. J Neurophysiol 1980;44:532–554.
27 Olszewski J: The Thalamus of the *Macaca mulatta*. An Atlas for Use with the Stereotaxic Instrument. Basel, Karger, 1952.
28 Wiesendanger R, Wiesendanger M: The thalamic connections with medial area 6 (supplementary motor cortex) in the monkey *(Macaca fascicularis)*. Exp Brain Res 1985;59:91–104.

Professor Katsuma Nakano, Department of Anatomy, School of Medicine,
Mie University, Tsu, Mie 514 (Japan)

Proceedings of the 2nd International Workshop on Microphysiological Recordings during Stereotactic Neurosurgery: Motor Thalamus, October 1–2, 1989, Nikko, Japan
Stereotact Funct Neurosurg 1993;60:62–69

Anatomical Distinctions between the Two Basal Ganglia Afferent Territories in the Primate Motor Thalamus[1]

Igor A. Ilinsky, Warren G. Tourtellotte, Kristy Kultas-Ilinsky

Department of Anatomy, University of Iowa College of Medicine, Iowa City, Iowa, USA

Key Words. Monkey · Motor thalamus · Nigral efferents · Pallidal efferents · PHA-L · Neuronal circuits

Abstract. In primates, the efferents of the two basal ganglia output structures, medial globus pallidus and substantia nigra pars reticularis, are completely segregated and target different thalamic regions. Despite similarities demonstrated earlier in non-primate species in the functional properties and ultrastructural features of the terminals of the two pathways, the present findings suggest significant differences between thalamic circuits associated with the two systems in primates. The data presented in this report further support the concept on functional and anatomical diversity of the subdivisions of the primate motor thalamus proposed in 1990 by Hinsky.

Introduction

Neuroanatomical studies have demonstrated that, in primates, the nigro- and pallidothalamic pathways are distributed to three subdivisions of the ventral thalamus without an overlap [1–4]. According to the latter two reports, nigrothalamic fibers terminate throughout the extent of the magnocellular subdivision of the ventral anterior nucleus (VAmc), while pallidothalamic fibers are topographically distributed to two other subdivisions of the same nucleus – densicellular (VAdc) and parvicellular (VApc). These findings are especially significant in view of the evidence indicating the existence of parallel circuits within the basal ganglia and their segregated output pathways via the thalamus to

[1] Supported by NIH research grant NS RO1 24188.

cortex. For example, one of these circuits [5–9] involves the caudate nucleus, which receives significant input from the prefrontal cortex and frontal eye fields and projects preferentially to the substantia nigra pars reticularis (SNr). The latter sends its axons to the VAmc as well as to the mediodorsal nucleus, and these thalamic nuclei project back to the same cortical areas [3, 10]. This multisynaptic circuit with the caudate as a processing and integration center of cortical and subcortical information can be associated with cognitive aspects of motor behavior, and it may constitute an anatomical substrate for control of visually sustained head and neck movements [11, 12]. Another multisynaptic basal ganglia circuit involves putamen as an integration center for information mostly from motor and somatosensory cortices with the output via the medial globus pallidus (GPm) and thalamus (VAdc and VApc) to the premotor and primary motor cortices [3, 13]. This circuit may be associated with the control of body and limb movements [14–16]. Although the two systems are connectionally distinct, they share a number of common features. For example, the striatal afferents to both GPm and SNr and the outputs from the latter are GABAergic and inhibitory [for references see 17, 18].

It is reasonable to assume that lesions in any part of the basal ganglia circuitry will, in one way or another, influence their outputs to the thalamus and eventually to the cortex. The available data on the organization of specific neuronal circuits associated with the basal ganglia outputs at the thalamic level are limited and controversial. The popular concept of a stereotype 'blueprint' of circuits common to all thalamic nuclei regardless of species and regional and functional differences [19, 20] has recently been challenged by ultrastructural studies in primates [21–23]. These results have pointed to fundamental differences in the synaptic and neuronal organization of nigral and cerebellar thalamic territories, and have demonstrated that neither was similar to sensory nuclei that have been analyzed in detail earlier [19, 24]. The present report will compare some general features of the organization of nigral and pallidal territories in the Rhesus monkey thalamus.

Materials and Methods

The study was performed on 7 adult Rhesus monkeys. The qualitative and quantitative neuroanatomical techniques used have been described in detail elsewhere [21].

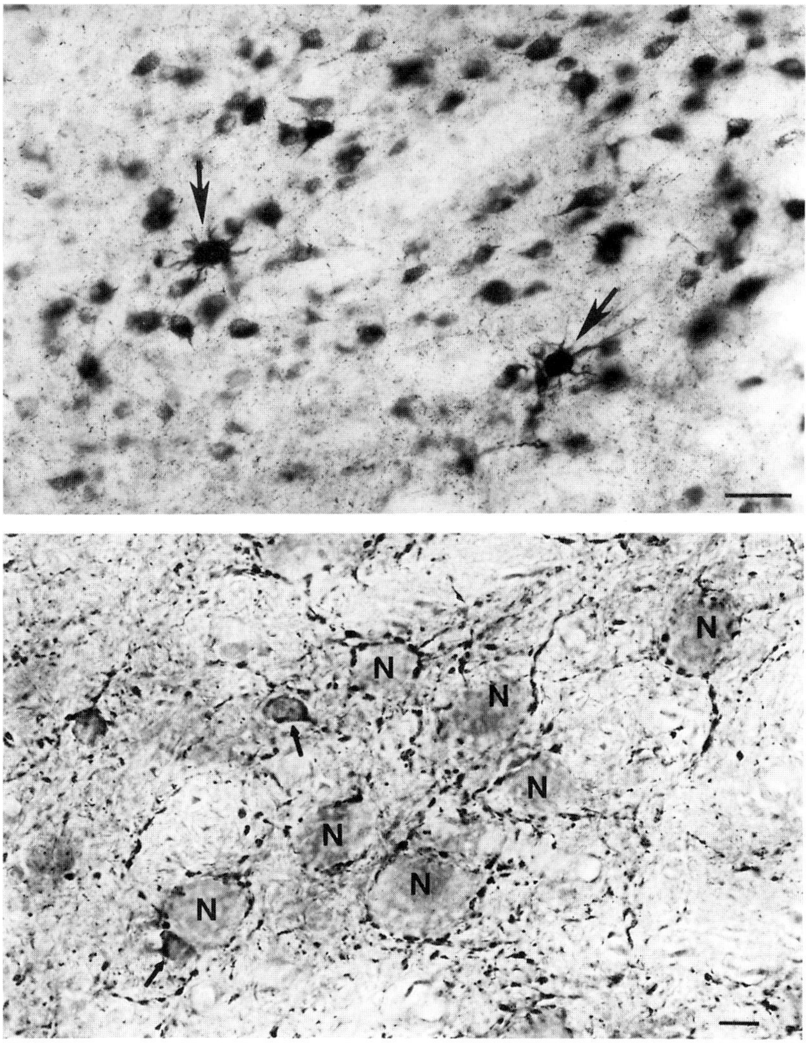

A

B

Fig. 1. Examples of cell clusters in the VAdc. **A** Retrogradely labeled cells after WGA-HRP injections in the motor cortex. Arrows point to two cell clusters with medium size neurons surrounded by smaller labeled cells. Labeling in the background is mostly due to the anterograde transport in corticothalamic fibers. Bar = 100 μm. **B** A cell cluster in a sagittal section stained for antibody to glutamic acid decarboxylase (GAD) viewed with phase-contrast illumination. Arrows point to two GAD immunoreactive LCN associated with this cluster. Somata of varying sizes unstained PN (N) are densely covered with GAD-positive boutons. Bar = 10 μm.

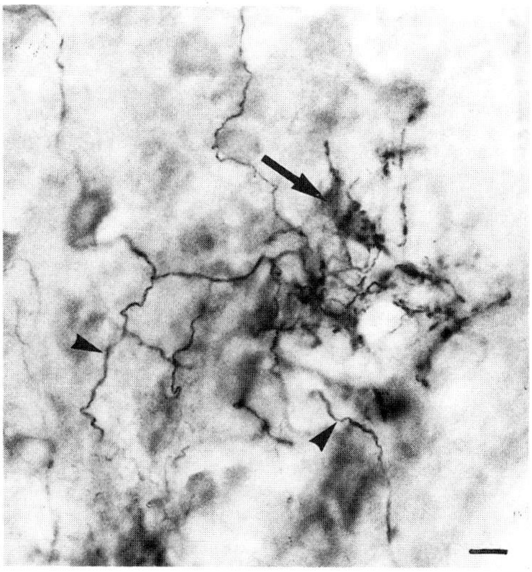

Fig. 2. An example of a dense plexus formed by pallidal fibers within a cell cluster. Pallidal fibers, have been labeled anterogradely after a PHA-L injection in the GPM. Several fibers (arrowheads) usually enter these clusters. The continuity of the fibers can be traced through consecutive focal planes. Arrow points to a cell densely covered with terminal enlargements of pallidal fibers. Bar = 10 μm.

Additional experiments described here were performed with the anterograde tracer *Phaseolus vulgaris* leukoagglutinin (PHA-L) injected iontophoretically into the GPm. The immunocytochemical procedure was according to Gerfen and Sawchenko [25].

Results

The neuronal and synaptic organization of the nigral projection zone in the monkey thalamus (VAmc) has been described in detail earlier [21, 22]. These studies have demonstrated that the VAmc is composed of two types of nerve cells: thalamocortical projection neurons (PN) and GABAergic local circuit neurons (LCN) that differ by their size and anatomical features. The VAmc cells appear to be distributed in random, without an apparent pattern. The nigral fibers from en-passant synapses on proximal dendrites and somata of PN and also contact LCN. The overall density of nigral boutons on PN somata is relatively low with most of the nigral input directed to their primary and secondary dendrites.

Unlike in the VAmc, cells in the VAdc comprising the major pallidal afferent territory of the thalamus are arranged in clusters and are

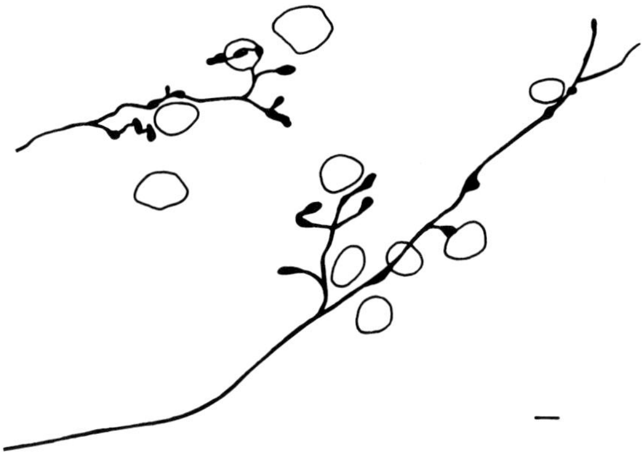

Fig. 3. Camera lucida drawings of two anterogradely labeled nigrothalamic fibers with their terminal ramifications. Some related neurons are shown with fine outline. Bar = 20 μm.

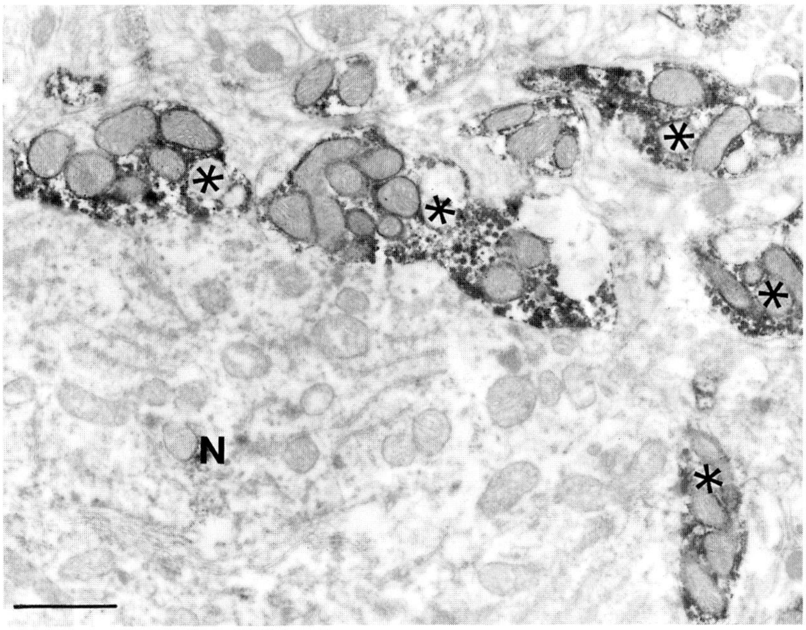

Fig. 4. An electronmicrograph illustrating numerous GAD immunoreactive axon terminals (asterisks) on a soma of a projection neuron (N) and in adjacent neurophil. Bar = 1 μm.

composed of two morphologically distinct types of PN, medium and small (fig. 1A). Each cluster contains also one or two GABAergic LCN (fig. 1B). Several pallidothalamic fibers target these cell clusters forming rather dense terminal pelxuses (fig. 2). A single pallidal fiber may contribute to plexuses in several cell clusters. This arrangement is different from that displayed by labeled nigrothalamic fibers, which do not form dense plexuses involving adjacent cells (fig. 3). Ultrastructurally, when identified with an autoradiographic label, pallidothalamic terminals are similar to nigral boutons; however, their density on somata of projection neurons is higher while the frequency of contacts on LCN is lower compared to nigrothalamic terminals in the VAmc. Consequently, the density of GABAergic boutons on PN somata in VAdc is very high (fig. 4).

According to our preliminary data, the corticothalamic inputs also appear to be differently organized in these two thalamic nuclei.

Discussion

The above brief comparison of the neuronal organization of pallidal and nigral afferent territories suggests that despite the general similarity in functional [26–28] and anatomical properties of nigral and pallidal efferents [29], the thalamic circuits that receive these inputs may differ in primates. This in turn implies different mechanisms for processing the activity from the two basal ganglia output systems and possibly functional differences in the thalamocortical pathways originating in the two regions.

In general, the synaptic organization of the nigrothalamic territory is relatively simple. A major unanswered question points to the overall functional significance of the nigrothalamic pathway, i.e., whether it regulates the dense corticothalamic input from the prefrontal cortex or whether its major role is to gate the ascending activity from the superior colliculus [21]. The latter connection has been demonstrated at the light-microscopic level [30], but ultrastructural details still need to be elucidated.

By contrast, the cell clusters found in the VAdc appear to represent the functional units in this nucleus. Future studies focusing upon the anatomical relationships within the clusters and the specific cortical targets of the two types of PN should provide greater understanding of this organization. Currently, it is apparent that thalamic circuits participating in the processing of efferent basal ganglia activity, funneled via globus pallidus, are more complex compared to those associated with the nigrothalamic pathway. This is consistent with the functional studies indicating involvement of GPm neurons in complex movements of the extremities [14], by contrast to the more stereotyped visually triggered head and neck movements with which the basal ganglia output via substantia nigra is believed to be associated [11].

References

1 Carpenter MB, Nakano K, Kim R: Nigrothalamic projections in the monkey demonstrated by autoradiographic techniques. J Comp Neurol 1976;165:401–416.

2 Kim R, Nakano K, Jayaraman A, Carpenter MB: Projections of the globus pallidus and adjacent structures: an autoradiographic study in the monkey. J Comp Neurol 1976;169:263–290.

3 Ilinsky IA, Jouandet ML, Goldman-Rakic PS: Organization of the nigrothalamocortical system in the rhesus monkey. J Comp Neurol 1985;236:315–330.

4 Ilinsky IA, Kultas-Ilinsky K: Sagittal cytoarchitectonic maps of the Macaca mulatta thalamus with a revised nomenclature of the motor-related nuclei validated by observations on their connectivity. J Comp Neurol 1987;262:331–364.

5 Yeterian EG, Van Hoesen GW: Cortico-striate projections in the Rhesus monkey: the organization of certain cortico-caudate connections. Brain Res 1978;139:43–63.

6 Van Hoesen GW, Yeterian EH, Lavizzo-Mourey R: Widespread corticostriate projections from temporal cortex of the Rhesus monkey. J Comp Neurol 1981;199: 205–219.

7 Selemon LD, Goldman-Rakic PS: Longitudinal topography and interdigitation of corticostriatal projections in the Rhesus monkey. J Neurosci 1985;5:776–794.

8 Selemon LD, Goldman-Rakic PS: Topographic intermingling of striatonigral and striatopallidal neurons in the Rhesus monkey. J Comp Neurol 1990;297:359–376.

9 Parent A, Bouchard C, Smith Y: The striatopallidal and striatonigral projections: Two distinct fiber systems in primate. Brain Res 1984;303:385–390.

10 Goldman-Rakic PS, Porrino LJ: The primate mediolateral (MD) nucleus and its projection to the frontal lobe. J Comp Neurol 1985;242:535–560.

11 DeLong MR, Crutcher MD, Georgopoulos AP: Relations between movement and single cell discharge in the substantia nigra of the behaving monkey. J Neurosci 1983;3:1599–1606.

12 Canavan AGM, Nixon PD, Passingham RE: Motor learning in monkeys *(Macaca fascicularis)* with lesions in motor thalamus. Exp Brain Res 1989;77:113–126.

13 Schell GR, Strick PL: The origin of thalamic inputs to the arcuate premotor and supplementary motor areas. J Neurosci 1984;4:539–560.

14 Georgopoulos AP, DeLong MR, Crutcher MD: Relations between parameters of step-tracking movements and single cell discharge in the globus pallidus and subthalamic nucleus of the behaving monkey. J Neurosci 1983;3:1586–1598.

15 DeLong MR, Crutcher MD, Georgopoulos AP: Primate globus pallidus and subthalamic nucleus: Functional organization. J Neurophysiol 1985;53:530–543.
16 Alexander GE, Crutcher MD: Neural representation of the target (goal) of visually guided arm movements in three motor areas of the monkey. J Neurophysiol 1990;64:164–178.
17 Kultas-Ilinsky K, Ilinsky IA: Neuronal and synaptic organization of the motor nuclei of mammalian thalamus; in Jones DG (ed): Current Topics in Research on Synapses. New York, Liss, 1986, vol 3, pp 77–145.
18 Reiner A, Anderson KD: The patterns of neurotransmitter and neuropeptide cooccurrence among striatal projection neurons: Conclusions based on recent findings. Brain Res Rev 1990;15:251–265.
19 Jones EG: The Thalamus. New York, Plenum Press, 1985.
20 Steriade M, Llinas RR: The functional states of the thalamus and the associated neuronal interplay. Physiol Rev 1988;68:649–742.
21 Ilinsky IA, Kultas-Ilinsky K: Fine structure of the magnocellular subdivision of the ventral anterior thalamic nucleus (VAmc) or *Macaca mulatta.* I. Cell types and synaptology. J Comp Neurol 1990;294:455–478.
22 Kultas-Ilinsky K, Ilinsky IA: Fine structure of the magnocellular subdivision of the ventral anterior thalamic nucleus (VAmc) of *Macaca mulatta.* II. Organization of nigrothalamic afferents as revealed with EM autoradiography. J Comp Neurol 1990;294:479–489.
23 Ilinsky IA: Structural and connectional diversity of the primate motor thalamus: Experimental light and electron microscopic studies in the Rhesus monkey. Stereotact Funct Neurosurg 1990;54/55:114–124.
24 Jones EG: Functional subdivision and synaptic organization of the mammalian thalamus. Int Rev Physiol Neurophysiol 1981;25:173–244.
25 Gerfen CR, Sawchenko PE: An anterograde neuroanatomical tracing method that shows the detailed morphology of neurons, their axons and terminals: Immunohistochemical localization of an axonally transported plant lectin. Phaseolus vulgaris leucoagglutinin (PHA-L). Brain Res 1984;290:219–238.
26 Yamamoto T, Hassler R, Huber C, Wagner A, Sasaki K: Electrophysiologic studies on the pallido- and cerebello-thalamic projections in squirrel monkeys *(Saimiri sciureus)*. Exp Brain Res 1983;51:77–87.
27 Uno M, Ozawa N, Yoshida M: The mode of pallidothalamic transmission investigated with intracellular recording from the cat thalamus. Exp Brain Res 1978; 33:493–507.
28 Ueki A: The mode of nigrothalamic transmission investigated with intracellular recording in the cat. Exp Brain Res 1983;49:116–124.
29 Kultas-Ilinsky K, Ilinsky IA, Warton A, Smith KR: Fine structure of nigral and pallidal afferents in the thalamus: An EM autoradiography study in the cat. J Comp Neurol 1983;216:390–405.
30 Harting JK, Huerta MF, Frankfurter AJ, Strominger NL, Royce GJ: Ascending pathways from the monkey superior colliculus: An autoradiographic analysis. J Comp Neurol 1980;192:853–882.

Igor A. Ilinsky, MD, PhD, Department of Anatomy, BSB 1–418,
University of Iowa College of Medicine, Iowa City, IA 52242 (USA)

Proceedings of the 2nd International Workshop on Microphysiological Recordings during Stereotactic Neurosurgery: Motor Thalamus, October 1–2, 1989, Nikko, Japan
Stereotact Funct Neurosurg 1993;60:70–79

Cerebello- and Pallido-Thalamic Pathways to Areas 6 and 4 in the Monkey

Kohnosuke Jinnai[a], *Atsushi Nambu*[b], *Ikuo Tanibuchi*[b], *Shin-ichi Yoshida*[b]

[a] Department of Physiology, Shiga University of Medical Sciences, Ohtsu, Shiga;
[b] Department of Integrative Brain Science, Faculty of Medicine, Kyoto University, Sakyo-ku, Kyoto, Japan

Key Words. Thalamus · Supplementary motor area · Premotor area · Arcuate premotor area · Cerebellar nucleus · Globus pallidus

Abstract. Projections from the cerebellar nuclei (CN) and the internal segment of the globus pallidus (GPi) to areas 6 and 4 via the thalamus were examined electrophysiologically in monkeys. In addition to the well-known pallido-thalamo-cortical projection to area 6, some thalamic neurons with CN input were found to project to area 6. Seventeen neurons in VLc, area X and the dorsal margin of VPLo were activated antidromically by stimulation of supplementary motor or premotor areas, and orthodromically by CN stimulation. Twelve neurons in area X and the medial part of VPLo were found to receive CN input and to project to the arcuate premotor area (APA). Four neurons in the VLo-X border region which were identified to project to APA were inhibited by GPi stimulation.

Introduction

It is well known that the cerebello-thalamic and pallido-thalamic projection fibers terminate in different regions of the ventral nuclear group. The former ends in VPLo, VLc and area X [1], while the latter ends in VLo and VApc [2]. The topographical organization of the thalamo-cortical projection implies that the cerebellar and basal ganglia output reach different areas of the cerebral cortex. For example, the cerebellar output is considered to project to the primary motor area, while the pallidal output projects to the supplementary motor and pre-

1011–6125/93/0603–0070 $ 2.75/0

motor areas [3, 4]. Recently, Nambu et al. [5] reported that the thalamic neurons receiving input from the internal segment of the globus pallidus (GP-thalamic neurons) project to the primary motor area. We [6, 7] also reported that the GP-thalamic neurons in VLo projecting to the arm region of the primary motor area show activity closely related with the movement of the upper limb. These findings suggest that both the cerebellar and the pallidal outputs are sent to the primary motor area and contribute to motor control activity. Our electrophysiological results are compatible with an anatomical report by Nakano et al. [8], which indicated the projection from VLo to the primary motor area, and with a recent report by Holsapple et al. [9]. These results raise the question whether the premotor and supplementary motor areas receive cerebellar input or not.

Methods

Two Japanese monkeys were prepared for the chronic experiment in which unitary activity of thalamic neurons were recorded during task performance. Under pentobarbital anesthesia, stimulating electrodes were implanted in the cerebellar nuclei (CN), internal segments of the globus pallidus (GPi), primary motor, premotor (rostral portion of dorsolateral area 6), supplementary motor (SMA) and arcuate premotor (APA) areas. A few months after the operation, a glass-coated Elgiloy microelectrode was inserted vertically into the thalamus to record unitary activity of single thalamic neurons. The cortical projection area of each thalamic neuron was determined by antidromic responses to stimulation of each area of the cerebral cortex (fig. 1). The inputs from the CN or from the GPi were examined by orthodromic discharges or suppression of spontaneous discharges of a thalamic neuron after stimulation of each structure. Details of the methods have already been described in previous papers [5, 7]. The discharge pattern of these thalamic neurons during task performance will be published later.

Results

Thalamic Neurons Projecting to SMA and the Premotor Area

Stimulation of SMA (intensity: usually less than 0.5 mA, single pulse of 0.3-ms duration) activated a considerably large number of thalamic neurons antidromically, and 48 were inhibited by GPi stimulation (0.5 mA, 0.3 ms). Time course of the inhibition was almost the same as in GP-thalamic neurons projecting to APA (fig. 1D, b) and of those projecting to the primary motor area [7].

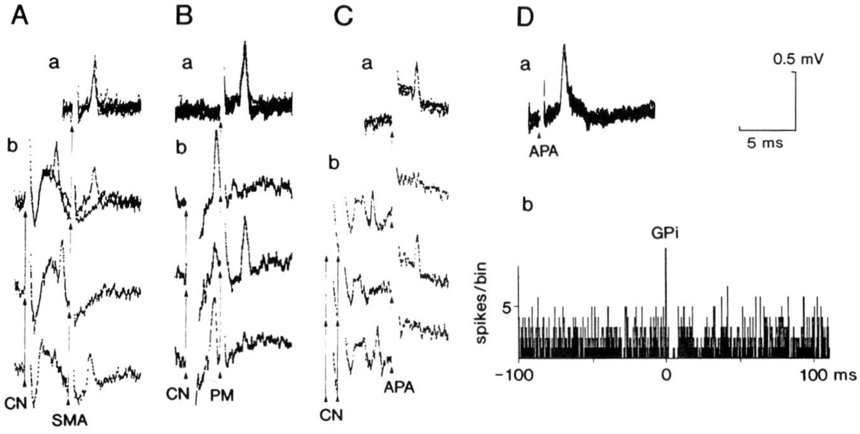

Fig. 1. Examples of CN-thalamic neurons projecting to (**A**) the supplementary motor (SMA); (**B**) premotor (PM); (**C**) arcuate premotor areas (APA), and (**D**) GP-thalamic neurons projecting to APA. a = Antidromic responses to stimulation of each cortical area. b in **A, B** and **C** = Orthodromic discharges elicited by CN stimulation and collision with antidromic responses. Calibration in **D** is applicable for all photograph recordings. Arrowheads indicate onset of CN and cortical stimulation. b in **D** = Post-stimulus time histogram showing the suppression of spontaneous discharges after GPi stimulation (sum of 150 sweeps, bin width; 0.5 ms).

Eleven thalamic neurons projecting to SMA were activated orthodromically by CN stimulation. Figure 1A shows an example of thalamic neurons with input from CN (CN-thalamic neurons). The locations of the SMA-stimulating electrodes which activated these neurons antidromically are illustrated in figure 2B, C. They were located within the area about 3.0 mm rostral to the caudal end of the arcuate sulcus. They also activated the GP-thalamic neurons antidromically. The threshold of antidromic response of these CN-thalamic neurons ranged from 0.2 to 0.7 mA, and was less than 0.5 mA in most neurons [9]. The stimuli with 0.5 mA intensity do not seem to spread effectively more than 1.5 mm, as discussed in previous reports (at this intensity, no single thalamic neuron was activated antidromically with both of the two cortical electrodes 3 mm apart from each other [5, 6]. Therefore, these antidromic responses cannot be due to current spread to the leg region of the primary motor area. The mean latency with SD of antidromic responses of CN-thalamic neurons (2.13 ± 0.71 ms) to SMA stimulation was significantly shorter than those of GP-thalamic neurons (3.74 ± 1.57 ms).

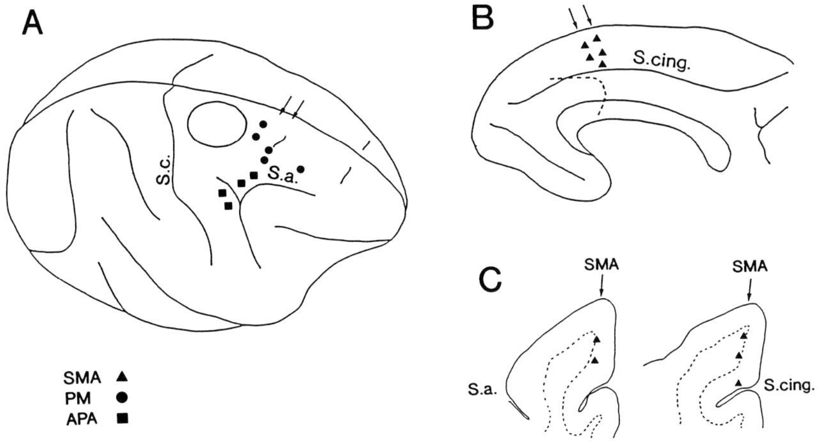

Fig. 2. Location of stimulating electrodes in area 6 of two monkeys, which activated both CN-thalamic and GP-thalamic neurons antidromically. **A** Electrodes in the arcuate premotor area (APA; squares) and the premotor area (PM; circles). Large oval shape indicates the position of the recording chamber. Arrows in **A, B** and **C** indicate the insertion points of the electrode arrays into SMA. **B** Tips of electrodes in the supplementary motor area (SMA; triangles). Dashed curve in **B** shows the approximate position of the arcuate sulcus. **C** The position of SMA electrode tips relative to cortical gray matter was illustrated on the coronal sections through the most ventral tip of each electrode array. S.c. = Central sulcus; S.a. = arcuate sulcus; S. cing. = cingulate sulcus.

The latency of the CN-induced discharge varied from 1.8 to 2.7 ms. The mean latency (2.35 ± 0.32 ms) of these responses was almost the same as that of CN-thalamic neurons projecting to the primary motor area (2.29 ± 0.67 ms), and was considered to be within the monosynaptic range. CN input to thalamic neurons was tested with 2.0 mA intensity of CN stimulation. The thresholds of CN-evoked discharges could be measured in 8 neurons, and were less than 0.5 mA in 5 neurons.

Twenty-eight thalamic neurons were activated antidromically by stimulation of the premotor area, of which 22 were inhibited by GPi stimulation. The other 6 thalamic neurons projecting to the premotor area were orthodromically activated by CN stimulation. Figure 1B shows an example of CN-evoked discharges of such neurons. Antidromic responses of these 6 neurons to stimulation of the premotor area had thresholds less than 0.5 mA. These responses were not due to current spread to APA, because four were elicited by electrodes far from APA and the other two were not activated by the most dorsal APA electrode (fig. 2A) The latency of CN-evoked discharges ranged from 2.0 to 4.0 ms. and was less than 2.8 ms in 5 cases. The threshold of CN-evoked discharges varied from 0.8 to 2.0 mA.

Thalamic Neurons Projecting to APA

Figure 1C shows an example of CN-thalamic neurons projecting to APA. Double shock stimulation of CN was necessary to activate this neuron at 0.5 mA intensity.

Twelve CN-thalamic neurons were antidromically activated by stimulation of APA with thresholds less than 0.5 mA. Five neurons were activated by the electrodes dorsal to the postarcuate spur which were far from the primary motor area, and the other 7 were activated by those ventral to the spur. Five of the latter were activated with current less than 0.14 mA. Therefore, most of these antidromic responses were not considered due to current spread to the primary motor area. Three of the latter were activated antidromically also by stimulation of the face region of the primary motor area with shorter latency and higher threshold than by APA stimulation. This indicated that the stimulation of the face region of the motor area activated the passing fibers or collateral branches of axons terminating in APA. The latency of CN-evoked discharges ranged from 1.9 to 3.2 ms, and was less than 2.7 ms in 10 neurons. The threshold of these responses was measured in 8 neurons, and was less than 0.6 mA in 6 neurons.

Five other thalamic neurons projecting to APA (4 were activated by electrodes in APA ventral to the spur) were inhibited by GPi-stimulation, as exemplified in figure 1D. Four of these neurons were found in the border region between VLo and area X. The threshold of these antidromic responses was less than 0.36 mA. These antidromic responses cannot be due to current spread to the premotor area because

---

Fig. 3. Location of GP-thalamic (white symbols) and CN-thalamic neurons (black symbols) projecting to the supplementary motor (SMA; triangles), premotor (PM; circles), arcuate premotor (APA; squares) and primary motor areas (Mot: + = GP-thalamic; dots = CN-thalamic neurons). White symbols with dots represent the neurons with both CN and GP input. CN = Cerebellar nuclei; GPi = internal segment of globus pallidus. Nomenclature and abbreviations of thalamic nuclei follow Olszewski [14]. Numerals indicate AP coordinates.

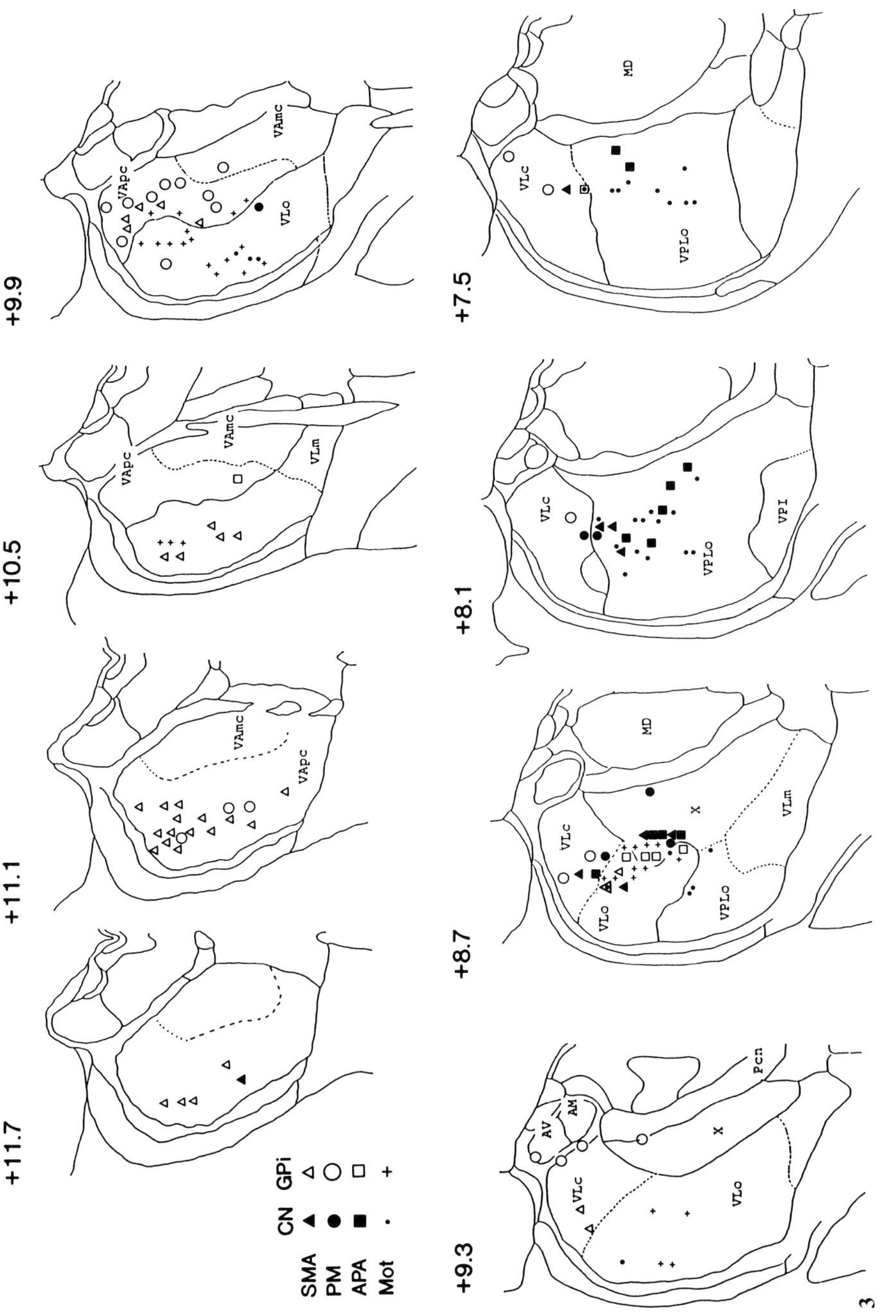
+11.7
+11.1
+10.5
+9.9
+9.3
+8.7
+8.1
+7.5
SMA PM APA Mot
CN GPi
VApc
VAmc
VLm
VLo
VLc
VPLo
VPI
MD
X
AV
AM
Pcn

3

their threshold is very low. Current spread to the frontal eye field is also not likely to activate these neurons, because projection from the border region between VLo and area X to area 8 has not been reported, and we did not see any thalamic neurons around this region which fired synchronously with eye movement.

Location of CN- and GP-Thalamic Neurons

Figure 3 shows the location of CN-thalamic and GP-thalamic neurons projecting to SMA, APA, premotor and primary motor areas. Several CN-thalamic and GP-thalamic neurons are not indicated here, because they could be tested only for either of the two inputs. CN-thalamic neurons projecting to SMA (black triangles) and premotor areas (black circles) are located mainly in the VLc, the dorsal margin of VPLo, and the dorsolateral part of area X. CN-thalamic neurons projecting to APA (black squares) are located mainly in the medial part of VPLo and area X. GP-thalamic neurons to APA (white squares) were found mainly in the border region between VLo and area X. GP-thalamic neurons projecting to SMA (white triangles) are located mainly in the VApc and the rostral portion of VLo. GP-thalamic neurons projecting to the premotor area (white circles) are distributed mainly in the dorsomedial part of VApc, but a few were found in the dorsal part of VLc. GP-thalamic neurons projecting to the primary motor area (plus symbols) were located mainly in VLo. CN-thalamic neurons to primary motor area are represented by dots.

Discussion

Our results indicate that a considerable number of CN-thalamic neurons project to the SMA and premotor areas. The threshold of CN stimulation for activating neurons was not measured in all the cases, but some of these thalamic neurons were activated by weak stimuli of less than 0.5 mA. In this study, thalamic neurons orthodromically activated by CN stimulation with current less than 2.0 mA were indicated to be CN-thalamic neurons. CN stimulation at this intensity does not seem to activate the neural structures in the dorsal part of the brain stem, because no sign of vestibulo-ocular or vestibulo-spinal reflexes (due to activation of vestibular nuclei) was observed, even with double shock stimuli at 2.0 mA. Furthermore, almost all of the CN-thalamic neurons projecting to these cortical areas were activated at rather fixed latencies of less than 2.8 ms, which are considered to be within the monosynaptic range. They were located in VLc, the dorsal margin of VPLo, and the dorsolateral portion of area X, where no ascending input from the brain stem other than CN has been reported [3]. Therefore, even if some structures in the brain stem might have been activated by CN stimulation, they would not have excited the thalamic neurons in these areas at a short and fixed latency.

The present electrophysiological data support an anatomical report by Wiesendanger and Wiesendanger [10] that injection of WGA-HRP into SMA resulted in retrograde transcellular labeling of cerebellar nuclei, probably via VLc and/or area X. Projection from these thalamic nuclei to the premotor area has also been reported by the same authors [11]. Input from CN to the premotor area has already been shown by the electrophysiological study by Sasaki et al. [12] that CN stimulation evoked field potentials in this cortical area. These observations join our present results to indicate that SMA and premotor area receive the input not only from GPi, but also from CN.

We found 12 CN-thalamic neurons projecting to APA, mostly in area X and the medial portion of VPLo. This finding coincides partially with the anatomical report by Schell and Strick [4] that projections to APA are mainly in area X. Several of these neurons in the medial part of VPLo were surrounded by neurons projecting to the face region of the primary motor area, and three were activated antidromically by stimulation of both the face region of the primary motor area and APA ventral to the postarcuate spur. This suggests a close relationship of APA to movement of the face. It is interesting to note the findings by Rizzolatti et al. [13] that many neurons in APA respond to visual presentation of objects around the mouth, or fire during arm movement toward the mouth.

Four GP-thalamic neurons, located in the border region between VLo and area X, were found to project to APA. The data indicated that APA also receives both CN and GPi inputs. Nakano et al. [8] reported that VApc, which is innervated by GPi, projected to layer I of APA. We also found one GP-thalamic neuron in VApc projecting to APA.

Recent anatomical and electrophysiological studies emphasize that the cerebellar and basal ganglia outputs terminate in separate regions of the cerebral cortex though the thalamus. This implies that the cerebellum and the basal ganglia work independently, and that they concern different kinds of motor control functions, e.g. control of movement in distal versus proximal musculature. Our previous report, however, showed that the outputs from both GPi and CN are relayed by the thalamus directly to the primary motor area [5, 6]. This was supported by a recent anatomical finding of Holsapple et al. [9] that the distal forelimb region of area 4 in the rostral bank of the central sulcus has strong projections from VLo, which receives GPi input, and moderately by VPLo. We consider that both the CN and GPi inputs are engaged at least in the control of distal forelimb movement.

The results in this paper indicate that rather wide regions of area 6, such as SMA, APA and the premotor area, also receive input from both CN and GPi through the thalamus. Therefore, interaction of the two inputs may occur in wide regions of area 4 and 6. It is probable that the cerebello-thalamo-cortical projection contributes not only to the activity of primary motor area, which controls movement in a direct manner, but also to the activity of area 6, which is related to more indirect control of movement, such as programming or preparatory process of movement.

Acknowledgements

The authors wish to thank Prof. K. Sasaki for careful review of the manuscript. Thanks are also due to Prof. T. Yokota for his constant encouragement.

References

1 Asanuma C, Thach WT, Jones EG: Anatomical evidence for segregated focal grouping of efferent cells and their terminal ramifications in the cerebello-thalamic pathway of the monkey. Brain Res Rev 1983;5:219–297.

2 Kim R, Nakano K, Jayaraman A, Carpenter MB: Projection of the globus pallidus and adjacent structures: An autoradiographic study in the monkey. J Comp Neurol 1976;169:263–290.

3 Jones EG: The Thalamus. New York, Plenum Press, 1985.

4 Schell GR, Strick PL: The origin of thalamic input to the arcuate premotor and supplementary motor areas. J Neurosci 1984;4:539–560.

5 Nambu A, Yoshida Y, Jinnai K: Projection on the motor cortex of thalamic neurons with pallidal input in the monkey. Exp Brain Res 1988;71:658–662.

6 Jinnai K, Nambu A, Yoshida Y: Activity of thalamic neurons conveying the basal ganglia output to the motor cortex; in Ito M (ed): Neural Programming. Taniguchi

Symposia on Brain Science, No 12. Tokyo, Japan Scientific Societies Press, 1989, pp 111–121.

7 Nambu A, Yoshida Y, Jinnai K: Movement related activities of thalamic neurons with input from the globus pallidus and projection to the motor cortex in the monkey. Exp Brain Res 1991, in press.

8 Nakano K, Kohno M, Hasegawa Y, Tokushige A, Sasaki K: Anatomical study of superficial and deep thalamocortical projection in the monkey. Neurosci Lett 1984;17(suppl):S64.

9 Holsapple JW, Preston JP, Strick PL: The origin of thalamic inputs to the 'hand' representation in the primary motor cortex. J Neurosci 1991, in press.

10 Wiesendanger R, Wiesendanger M: Cerebellocortical linkage in the monkey as revealed by transcellular labeling with the lecitin wheat germ agglutinin conjugated to the marker horseradish peroxidase. Exp Brain Res 1985;59:105–117.

11 Wiesendanger M: Organization of secondary motor areas of cerebral cortex; in Brooks (ed): Handbook of Neurophysiology. The Nervous System II: Motor Control. Washington, American Physiological Society, 1981, pp 1121–1147.

12 Sasaki K, Kawaguchi S, Oka H, Sakai M, Mizuno N: Electrophysiological studies on the cerebellocerebral projections in monkeys. Exp Brain Res 1976;24:495–507.

13 Rizzolatti G, Scandolara C, Matelli C, Gentilucci M: Afferent properties of periarcuate neurons in Macaque monkeys. 2. Visual responses. Behav Brain Res 1981;2:147–163.

14 Olszewski J: The Thalamus of the *Macaca mulatta*. An Atlas for Use with the Stereotaxis Instrument. Basel, Karger, 1952.

Dr. Kohnosuke Jinnai, Department of Physiology,
Shiga University of Medical Sciences, Ohtsu, Shiga 520–21 (Japan)

Proceedings of the 2nd International Workshop on Microphysiological Recordings during Stereotactic Neurosurgery: Motor Thalamus, October 1–2, 1989, Nikko, Japan
Stereotact Funct Neurosurg 1993;60:80

Levodopa-Induced Dyskinesia and Thalamotomy

H. Narabayashi, T. Yokochi, Y. Nakajima
Tokyo, Japan

Due to the accumulated experience with levodopa therapy, several authors have pointed out that levodopa-induced dyskinesia (DID) does not appear on the previously operated side. We intend to analyze which structure is responsible for this phenomenon.

A retrospective study classified the cases with DID operated unilaterally into three groups: (a) relatively large lesion involving both the VL and the V.im (mostly before 1972 not using the microelectrode technique) in the pre-dopa era; (b) very small lesion within the V.im aiming to control only tremor (with the microelectrode technique) leaving rigidity to pharmacotherapy, and (c) two lesions on the V.im and the VL (using the microelectrode technique). Satisfactory control or elimination of DID was observed only in the case of (a) and (c) and not (b). In (b), DID was controlled much less or only transiently.

It is concluded that DID was eliminated when VL was lesioned and that DID is the phenomenon depending on the pallido-thalamic (VL) projection and not on the V.im. DID is therefore interpreted as a reverse phenomenon of rigidity, both depending on the same structures, i.e. the pallidothalamic projection system, which is under inhibitory control by the striatum.

It is advised that microelectrode stereotactic VL thalamotomy is useful when DID is the disturbing factor for continuation of long-term levodopa therapy.

1011–6125/93/0603–0080 $ 2.75/0

Proceedings of the 2nd International Workshop on Microphysiological Recordings during Stereotactic Neurosurgery: Motor Thalamus, October 1–2, 1989, Nikko, Japan
Stereotact Funct Neurosurg 1993;60:81–85

Stereotactic Thalamotomy for Dystonic Patients

Katsumi Yamashiro[a], *Ronald R. Tasker*[b]

[a] Department of Neurosurgery, Nagasaki University School of Medicine, Nagasaki, Japan; [b] Department of Neurosurgery, University of Toronto, Canada

Key Words. Dystonia · Thalamotomy · Stereotactic surgery · Ventral intermediate nucleus · Posterior ventral oral nucleus

Abstract. A total of 54 patients (22 females and 32 males) with dystonia underwent thalamotomy. These patients consisted of 25 dystonia musculorum deformans (DMD) and 29 secondary dystonia cases. All of the patients were analyzed prospectively. Preoperative and postoperative symptoms were compared and grade. The target areas of thalamotomy were the ventral intermediate (Vim) and posterior ventral oral (Vop) nuclei. 59% of the patients showed more than 25% improvement, 23% were slightly improved cases (less than 25%), and 16% showed no change or their symptoms had worsened.

Introduction

Surgical treatment for dystonia has been reported by many authors and includes many target areas [1–13], but has shown variable results.

In relation to stereotactic thalamotomy, the largest series has been reported by Cooper [4–6] who operated on 227 patients with dystonia, and summarized his experience after a mean follow-up period of 7.9 years. 69.7% of the patients showed improvement after stereotactic surgery. We describe here the results of stereotactic thalamotomy in 54 cases of generalized dystonia, both dystonia musculorum deformans (DMD) and secondary dystonia.

1011–6125/93/0603–0081 $ 2.75/0

Materials and Methods

A total of 54 patients (22 females and 32 males) with dystonia were operated on between 1961 and 1985 by the senior author (RRT). Data on all the patients were analyzed prospectively [12]. Twenty-nine patients were classified as secondary dystonia, 8 due to birth injury, 9 to postnatal head injury, 4 to encephalitis, 1 to birth injury and encephalitis, 1 to meningitis, 1 to hemolytic disease, 1 to subarachnoid hemorrhage, 2 to stroke, 1 to anoxia, and 1 due to unknown cause. Twenty-five DMD patients were classified into 8 familial, 12 nonfamilial, and 5 retarded children. Data were compared between the last review prior to the first stereotactic operation performed (preoperative review) and the most recent review recorded postoperatively (postoperative review), by recording the average grade change for each group of patients. The operation was performed in the standard fashion by techniques described previously [11, 12] with the target in the ventral intermediate (Vim) or posterior ventral oral (Vop) nucleus of the thalamus about 14–15 mm lateral from the midline. The physiological localization was accomplished using macrostimulation until 1982, and after that by microrecording and microstimulation [12]. A few early lesions were made using a small leukotome or a cryoprobe by a 1.1-mm in diameter with 3-mm bare tip electrode. Radiofrequency lesion size was about 3–5 mm, and that of the cryoprobe was about 4–7 mm in diameter. When a single lesion was not effective, an additional lesion was made.

Each patient target and estimated lesion size were plotted on a standard brain map.

Results

Thalamotomies were done on the right side in 19 patients, on the left side in 19, and on both sides in 16. In the primary dystonia group, the number of operations on the right side was higher than that for the left side. On the other hand, the secondary dystonia group showed a larger number on the left side, but not with a statistically significant difference.

The site of the targets was drawn from the operation records (fig. 1), which include not only the first operative results, but also those for the second and third operations. Both the primary and the secondary groups showed that the most frequent target sites were in the Vim and then in the Vop nucleus. A few lesions were made in the ventralis caudalis nucleus (Vc), the internal capsule (IC), and in the anterior ventral oral nucleus (Voa). There were no lesions in the centrum medianum (CM) nucleus. The relationship between the efficacy and the thalamotomy site of primary DMD cases is shown in figure 2. In excellent cases (improved more than 50% of preoperative assessment in our grading), lesions were made in Vim and Vop. Those affected areas

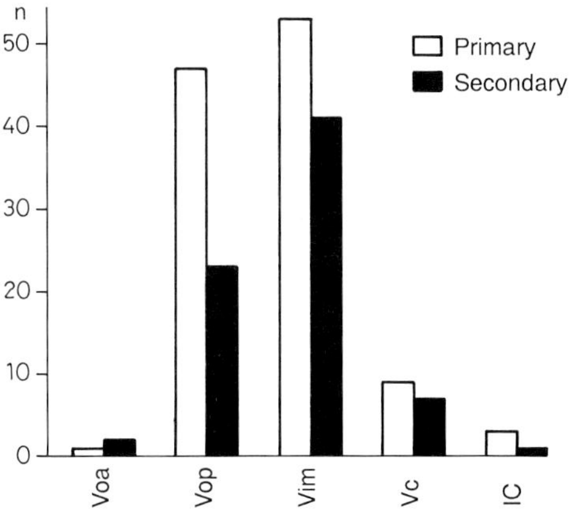

Fig. 1. Target sites during stereotactic operation in dystonic patients.

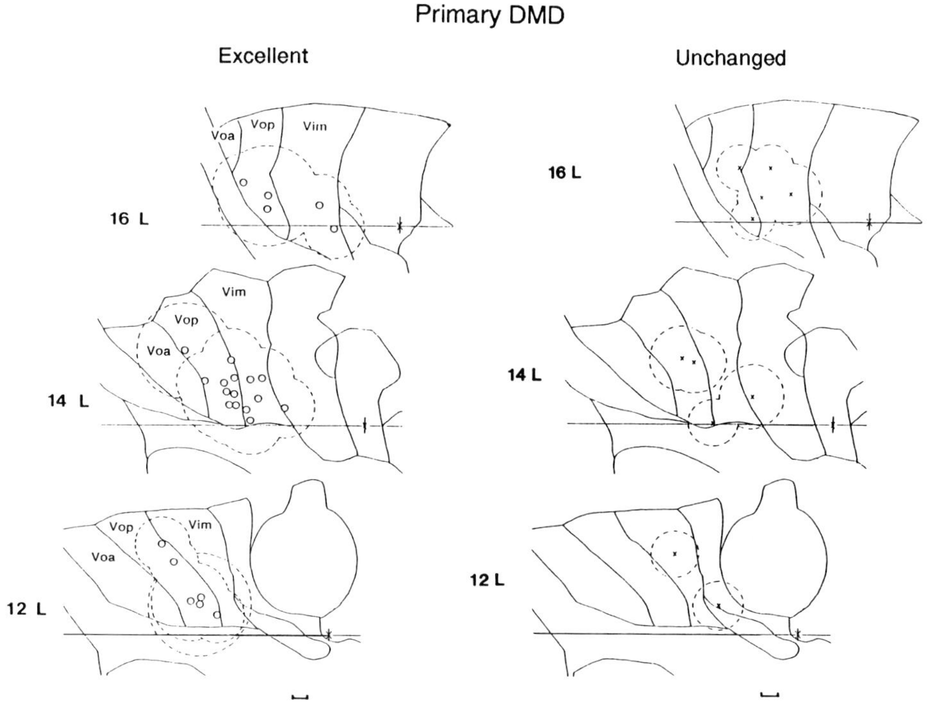

Fig. 2. Relationship between efficacy and thalamotomy sites in DMD cases.

expanded to rostral and dorsal, sometimes to Voa and IC, but did not extend to the CM or subthalamic nucleus (sub Th). On the other hand, the unchanged cases showed less expansion rostrally when compared to the excellent cases. Most of lesion of Vc were seen in the unchanged cases, and also small size lesions in the medial plane.

The results of all thalamotomies were as follows: 34% were more than 50% improved, 25% were moderately (25–50%) improved, 23% were slightly (less than 25%) improved, and 16% showed no change or were worse. Especially, retarded DMD cases showed good improvement.

Discussion

The etiology of DMD is not totally known. Secondary dystonia has etiologies, such as association with other hereditary neurological symptoms or peripheral cerebral injury, infection, head trauma, stroke, and brain tumor [14].

Many targets were selected for surgical treatment of dystonia, such as the internal capsule [14], dentate nucleus [13], cerebral peduncle [8], putamen [15], subthalamus [7], pulvinar [4–6], Vim, VL, CM, ventrocaudal (Vc) thalamic nuclei, and combinations of those [4–7]. In general, the target for thalamotomy was Vim, VL, CM and Vc of thalamic nuclei and the pulvinar and posterior lateral (LP) complex. Cooper's [4–6] target was usually the center of the posterior half of the VL and CM nuclei. Bertrand et al. [2] also reported lesions in that almost the same area where the VL lesion was made.

Improvement was seen in 69.7% of posterior VL thalamotomies [4–6], 35% of anterior VL thalamotomies [3], 25% of Vim, Vc and CM lesions [1], 50% of CM lesions [9], and 67% of thalamo-subthalamotomies [7]. We selected the Vim and Vop nuclei as the target sites for treatment of both primary and secondary dystonia, and our results showed that larger lesions in the Vim and Vop nuclei produced good clinical improvement.

References

1 Andrew J, Fowler CJ, Harrison MSG: Stereotaxic thalamotomy in 55 cases of dystonia. Brain 1983;106:981–1000.
2 Bertrand C, Molina-Negro P, Martinez SN: Stereotaxic targets for dystonia and dyskinesias: Relationship to corticobulbar fibers and other adjoining structures. Adv Neurol 1979;24:395–399.
3 Carcalos A: Results of 103 cryosurgical procedures in involuntary movement disorders. Confin Neurol 1972;34:74–81.
4 Cooper IS: Dystonia: Surgical approaches to treatment and physiological implications; in Yahr MD (ed): The Basal Ganglia. New York, Raven Press, 1976, pp 369–383.
5 Cooper IS: 20-year follow-up study of the neurosurgical treatment of dystonia musculorum deformans. Adv Neurol 1976;14:423–453.
6 Cooper IS: Dystonia; in Schaltenbrand G, Walker AE (eds): Stereotaxy and the Human Brain. Stuttgart, Thieme, 1982, pp 545–561.
7 Gros G, Frerebeau PH, Perez-Dominguez E, Bazin M, Privat JM: Long-term results of stereotaxic surgery for infantile dystonia and dyskinesia. Neurochirurgia 1976;19:171–178.
8 Maspes PE Pagni CA: Surgical treatment of dystonia and choreoathetosis in infantile cerebral palsy by pedunculotomy. Pathological observation and therapeutic results. J Neurosurg 1964;21:1076–1086.
9 Ramamurthi B, Davidson A: Central median lesions-analysis of 89 cases. Confin Neurol 1975;37:63–72.
10 Taira T, Hitchcock E: Stereotactic thalamotomy for patients with dystonia. Stereotact Funct Neurosurg 1990;54/55:215–216.
11 Tasker RR, Organ LW, Hawrylyshyn P: The Thalamus and Midbrain of Man: A Physiological Atlas Using Electrical Stimulation. Springfield, Thomas, 1982.
12 Tasker RR, Doorly T, Yamashiro K: Thalamotomy in generalized dystonia. Adv Neurol 1988;50:615–631.
13 Zervas NT: Long-term review of dentatectomy in dystonia musculorum deformans and cerebral palsy. Acta Neurochir 1974;24:49–51.
14 Fahn S: Concept and classification of dystonia. Adv Neurol 1988;50:1–8.
15 Demiere B, Rondolt P: Dystonia caused by putamino-capsulo-caudate vascular lesions. J Neurol Neurosurg Psychiatr 1983;46:404–409.
16 Heimburger RF: Putamectomy as an aid to upper extremity control. Confin Neurol 1975;37:16–23.

Katsumi Yamashiro, MD, Department of Neurosurgery, Nagasaki University School of Medicine, 7–1 Sakamoto-machi, Nagasaki 852 (Japan)

Proceedings of the 2nd International Workshop on Microphysiological Recordings during Stereotactic Neurosurgery: Motor Thalamus, October 1–2, 1989, Nikko, Japan
Stereotact Funct Neurosurg 1993;60:86–93

Unit Activity of Nucleus Ventralis lateralis of Human Thalamus during Voluntary Movements

S.N. Raeva

Chemical Physics Institute of the Academy of Sciences, Burdenko Neurosurgery Institute of the USSR Academy of Medical Sciences, Moscow, Russia

Key Words. Human thalamus · Ventralis lateralis neuron · Microelectrode recording · Voluntary movement · Stereotactic surgery

Abstract. The dynamics of change of single VL neurons of human thalamus during voluntary movements was investigated in the course of stereotactic operations on dyskinetic patients. Two basic types of units (A and B cells), reacting to the voluntary movement with different discharge patterns, revealed the common dynamics and a transient time-connectivity of responses correlated with certain phases of the performance of motor acts. It is supposed that these findings reflect the dynamic conjugation of two functionally different cellular subsystems in the human thalamus, which perform collaborative processing and transmitting of information during voluntary movements.

Introduction

The results of microelectrode recording and of macro- and microstimulation in the human VL and Vim thalamic nuclei in parkinsonism and related disorders offer the opportunity to study mechanisms of voluntary and involuntary movements [1–10]. The aim of the present study was to analyze the firing patterns and functional properties of VL neurons as well as to reveal the mechanism of processing and transmitting information by these elements during voluntary movements in man.

1011–6125/93/0603–0086 $ 2.75/0

Materials and Methods

The activity of 228 single neurons of the VL was recorded extracellularly with tungsten microelectrodes (resistance 1–2 mΩ) in the course of 36 stereotactic operations (surgeons A. Kadin, N. Vasin, V. Shabalov, N. Grochovsky). Basic methods of recording and analysis were similar to those described in our previous studies [7, 8]. Monopolar recording was used. The surface EEG, EMG of the tested limbs and the phonogram were recorded simultaneously with the spike discharges. Microelectrode trajectories from the premotor cortex toward the VL were monitored with X-rays. Operations were performed under local anesthesia. Several voluntary motor tests performed in response to verbal commands such as 'Clench your hand!' and 'Unclench!' were used. Passive movements and tactile stimuli were applied as well. The alterations of neuronal changes and EMG activities correlating with functionally different phases of voluntary movement (preparation and initiation, movement realization, after effect) were analyzed with computer techniques.

Results

The quantitative analysis of the background and evoked activity of Voa-Vop units showed that the VL neurons could be classified into two basic types of elements (A and B cells) characterized by differences in their discharge patterns and functional properties.

The spontaneous pattern of A units (171 of 228, 75%) was represented by irregular unitary discharges varying between 3 and 20 per second. As can be seen in figure 1, the interspike interval histogram shows the Poisson-like distribution with wide dispersion. The autocorrelation histogram and spectral density show the absence of regularity in spike discharges. According to our previous data [7–9], one of the essential peculiarities of this type of VL cells was a tendency of discharges to modify irregular nonrhythmic activity into a transient quasi-rhythmic one in the range of 4–6 Hz, which visibly increased during or after the performance of motor tests (50%).

The spontaneous pattern of B units (57 of 228, 25%), unlike A cells, was represented by short (duration 7–20 ms) burst rhythmic discharges in the range of 3–6 Hz (fig. 1). The intraburst interval histogram was characterized by high stability; its dispersion was narrow. The interburst interval varies in different cells in the range of 150–250 ms. The autocorrelation histograms and spectral density of B units, contrary to A cells, showed regularity of spike burst rhythmic discharges. The cross-correlation histograms do not reveal any connection be-

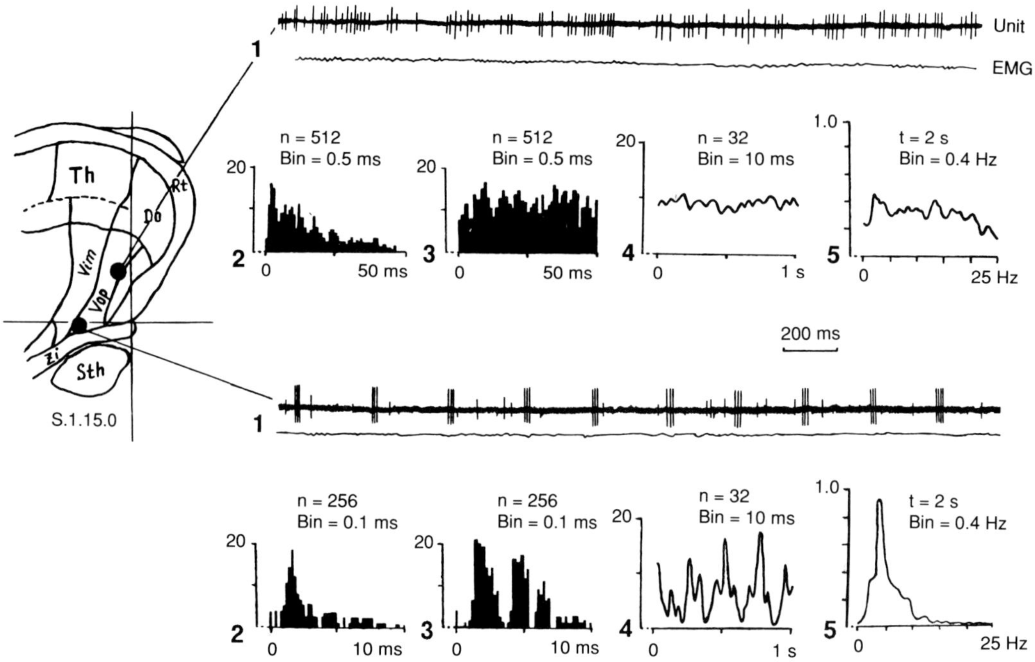

Fig. 1. Spontaneous firing pattern of irregular unitary spike activity of A-type neurons (above) and burst rhythmic discharges of B-type neurons (below) in the nucleus VL of the human thalamus.

Left: The scheme of human deep structures of the atlas by Schaltenbrand and Bailey [1959]. Right: 1 = unit activity (Unit) and electromyogram (EMG) of contralateral finger flexors; 2 = interspike interval histogram; 3 = autocorrelation histogram, n = number of coincidences (intraburst interval for B unit); 4 = autocorrelation function, n = number of coincidences-frequency (Hz); 5 = spectral density, abscissa-frequency (Hz), ordinate-units of dispersion.

tween the rhythmic activity of B units and the parkinsonian tremor. The existence of this type of bursting cells in akinetico-rigid parkinsonian, torticollis and cerebral palsy patients without tremor (or under general anesthesia) described in the literature [3, 4], and our data [7–9], suggests that this type of rhythmic activity in the VL is not of a pathological nature.

Figure 2 presents the typical changes in activity of responsive A and B neurons recorded simultaneously and EMG data during the performance of voluntary movements.

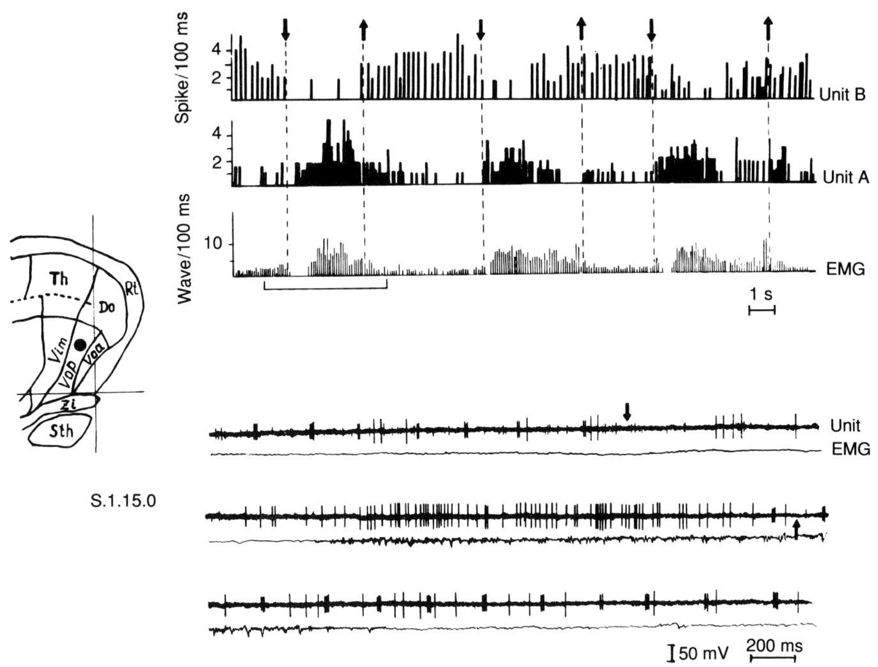

Fig. 2. The reactions of simultaneously recorded A and B units and EMG changes during the performance of three similar motor tasks in parkinsonian patient.

Left: The scheme of human deep structures. Above: Firing rate histogram of A and B units and EMG of finger flexors. The solid line under the lower image delimits the time interval during which lower traces were taken. Below: The unit activity and EMG. The arrows mark the presentation of commands 'Clench your hand!', 'Unclench!'.

The moment of preparation and the initial part of movement is accompanied by the appearance of tonic (duration 1.0–3.0 s) activatory reaction of A unit (102 of 155, 66%) and of reciprocal prolonged, inhibitory reaction of B unit (46 of 56, 82%). The termination of the movement is accompanied by the reverse patterns occurring as a rebound effect in the form of transient co-activation of A and B cells. This coactivation is represented in A cells by the appearance of the abovementioned tendency of discharges to modify their nonrhythmic activity into a quasi-rhythmic one at the frequency of about 5 Hz, and in B cells

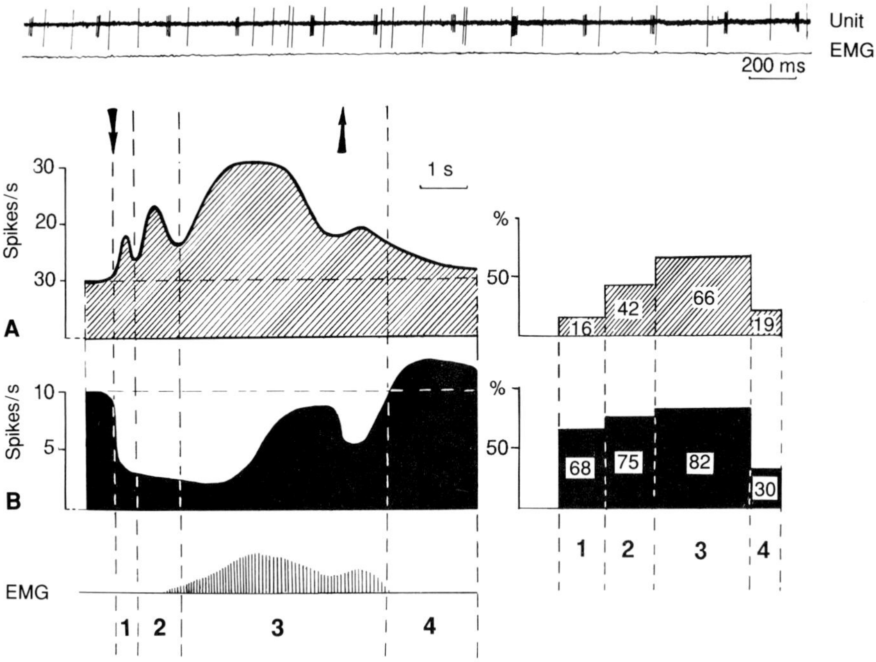

Fig. 3. The averaged dynamics of A and B unit responses and EMG changes during four fonctionally different phases of voluntary movements: (1) presentation; (2) preparation and movement initiation; (3) movement realization, and (4) after effect.

Above: The unit activity and EMG of finger flexors. Below left: average parameters of changes of A (A) and B (B) units and electromyogram (EMG); below right: percentage of the total quantity of A and B units responding during different phases of voluntary movements. The arrows mark the presentation of commands 'Clench your hand!', 'Unclench!'.

by the stabilization of rhythmicity in the range of 4–5 Hz. The activatory response pattern of A cells was observed during the performance of a wide range of voluntary movements of the upper and lower limbs, expressed more intensively on the contralateral side. Certainly, these cells are the 'voluntary movement' cells [2]. Unlike A cells, the typical evoked inhibitory pattern of B cells was observed not only during voluntary movements but also in response to different functional tests (passive joint movements, opening and closing of the eyes, command presentation, etc.) as well.

Figure 3 presents the general statistical evaluation of averaged dynamics of A and B types of unit responses and EMG changes during four functionally different phases of our basic model of voluntary movements: (1) command presentation; (2) preparation and initiation; (3) movement realization; (4) after effect. The data show a common cooperative character of interaction between A and B units in the VL and a transient time-connectivity of reactions, correlated with definite phases of the performance of voluntary movements. The preparation and initial part of movement are accompanied by the appearance of reciprocal conjugated response patterns of A and B cells: the appearance of tonic activations of A units and of prolonged inhibitory reactions of B units. The height of muscular contraction is accompanied by the reverse discharge patterns. The latter occurs in the form of the above-mentioned transient co-activation of A and B cells with a tendency to fire in common quasi-rhythmic discharges at a frequency of about 5 Hz. The dynamics of interrelation between these types of elements in the human VL during voluntary motor acts was described in detail in our previous paper [11].

The analysis of the functional features of neurons located not only in the VL, but in the nucleus reticularis thalami and some other thalamic nuclei [8] leads to the suggestion that the populations of these two (A, B) basic elements reflect the dynamic conjugation of two functionally different cellular subsystems in the human thalamus. These two subsystems probably interact as a common regulatory mechanism performing collaborative processing and transmitting of both afferent and efferent influences during voluntary movements [9–11]. One gets the impression that while A-cell populations appear to transmit signal messages, B-cell populations seem to facilitate this transmission by means of modulating activity levels and frequency filtration.

The essential functional differences between A and B neurons manifest themselves by different spontaneous (fig. 1) and evoked (fig. 2) patterns as well as by their reactivity to applied stimulation (fig. 3). The latter is demonstrated by different numbers of A and B units reacting to functionally different phases of a voluntary motor act. This fact indicates that the polyfunctional nature of B cells in the VL has a different, more nonspecific nature as compared to that of A units. It is noteworthy that B cells may scarcely be connected directly with somatic afferent inflows during voluntary movement. Taking into account the characteristics of B units and their participation in inhibitory processes, we think that the B type of VL neurons in the human thalamus resembles the so-called reticular cells or intrinsic thalamic interneurons of the inhibitory type [12–14]. In this respect our suggestion correlates with the data observed in the nucleus ventralis intermedius [3, 4] and in the nucleus reticularis [10] of the human thalamus. We suppose that these inhibitory processes dynamically sculpture spatial integrative patterns of neuronal activity in the course of voluntary movement and play a very important role in the genesis of pathological tremor.

Acknowledgements

The author thanks her collegues Dr. N. Wainberg and Dr. W. Dubinin for their great assistance with the statistical analysis.

References

1 Albe-Fessard D, Guiot G, Lammare Y, et al: Activation of thalamocortical projections related to tremorgenic processes; in Purpura DP, Yahr MD (eds): The Thalamus. New York, Columbia University Press, 1966, pp 237–253.
2 Jasper H, Bertrand G: Thalamic units involved in somatic sensation and voluntary and involuntary movements in man; in Purpura DP, Yahr MD (eds): The Thalamus. New York, Columbia University Press, 1966, pp 365–390.
3 Ohye Ch, Saito Y, Fukamachi A, et al: An analysis of the spontaneous rhythmic and non-rhythmic burst discharges in the human thalamus. J Neurol Sci 1974; 22:245–259.
4 Ohye Ch, Albe-Fessard D: Rhythmic discharges related to tremor in humans and monkeys; in Chalazonitis N, Boisson M (eds): Abnormal Neuronal Discharges. New York, Raven Press, 1978, pp 37–48.
5 Ohye Ch, Narabayashi H: Physiological study of presumed ventralis intermedius neurons in the human thalamus. J Neurosurg 1979;50:290–297.
6 Lenz F, Tasker R, Kwan H, et al: Single unit analysis of the human ventral thalamic nuclear group: Correlation of thalamic 'tremor cells' with the 3–6 Hz component of parkinsonian tremor. J Neurosci 1988;8:754–764.
7 Raeva S: Unit activity of some deep nuclear structures of the human brain during voluntary movements; in Somjen G (ed): Neurophysiology Studied in Man. Amsterdam, Excerpta Medica, 1972, pp 69–78.
8 Raeva S: Localization in human thalamus of units triggered during 'verbal commands', voluntary movements and tremor. Electroencephalogr Clin Neurophysiol 1986;63:160–173.
9 Raeva S: Unit activity of the human thalamus during voluntary movements. Stereotact Funct Neurosurg 1990;54-5:154–158.

10 Raeva S, Lukashev A, Lashin A: Unit activity in nucleus reticularis of human thalamus. Electroencephalogr Clin Neurophysiol 1992, in press.
11 Raeva S, Dubinin V, Wainberg N: A model of thalamic dynamic neuronal microsystems proving voluntary movements in man; in Holden A, Kryukov V (eds): Neurocomputers and Attention. Oxford Road, Manchester University Press, in press.
12 Jones E: The Thalamus. New York, Plenum Press, 1985.
13 Shosaku: Cross-correlation analysis of recurrent inhibitory circuits in the rat thalamus. J Neurophysiol 1986;55:1030–1043.
14 Sumitomo I, Takahashi Y, Kayama Y, Ogawa T: Burst discharges associated with phasic hyperpolarising oscillations of rat ventrobasal relay neurons. Brain Res 1988;466:354–362.

S.N. Raeva, MD, Laboratory of Human Cell Neurophysiology,
Institute of Chemical Physics, Academy of Sciences, Kosygin Street 4,
117977 Moscow (Russia)

Proceedings of the 2nd International Workshop on Microphysiological Recordings during Stereotactic Neurosurgery: Motor Thalamus, October 1–2, 1989, Nikko, Japan
Stereotact Funct Neurosurg 1993;60:94–103

Role of the Thalamus in Parkinsonian Tremor: Evidence from Studies in Patients and Primate Models

F.A. Lenz[a], *J.L. Vitek*[a], *M.R. DeLong*[b]

[a] Department of Neurosurgery, Johns Hopkins University, Baltimore, Md.,
[b] Department of Neurology, Emory University, Atlanta, Ga., USA

Key Words. Thalamus · Parkinson's disease · Tremor · Basal ganglia · Neuronal oscillators · Feedback processes

Abstract. The electrophysiologic basis of parkinsonian tremor is discussed in terms of the central oscillator and peripheral feedback hypotheses of tremor. Recent studies in monkeys and humans suggest that parkinsonian tremor may result from the activity of a central oscillator, possibly located in the basal ganglia. Peripheral somatosensory input seems to modulate tremor and central nervous system activity related to tremor.

Introduction

Two general models have been proposed to explain the mechanism of parkinsonian tremor – the central oscillator and peripheral feedback hypotheses [1–6]. The central oscillator hypothesis suggests that tremor results from the activity of central pacemaker cells independent of inputs from the periphery. By contrast, the peripheral hypothesis suggests that tremor results from oscillation of feedback circuit(s) in somewhat the same way as clonus results from the activity of an unstable spinal reflex feedback circuit.

Several facts link the 3–6 Hz component of resting tremor in Parkinson's disease with thalamic nuclei ventralis intermedius (Vim) and ventralis oralis posterior (Vop) [nomenclature of Hassler, ref. 7, see discussion in refs. 8, 9]. Many neurons in presumed Vim and Vop of parkinsonian patients show a large amount of tremor frequency activity that is correlated with tremor (tremor-related activity), as demonstrated by spectral analysis [10]. The timing of tremor-related activity relative to tremor is consistent with its involvement in the generation of tremor [11]. Finally, a small lesion involving presumed Vim or Vop, or both, relieves parkinsonian tremor [12]. This paper explores the extent to which the available data support the central oscillator or peripheral feedback hypotheses of thalamic tremor-related activity.

Central Oscillator Hypothesis

Thalamic Oscillators Potentially Involved in Tremor

Thalamic neurons function in two basic modes: the transfer mode and oscillatory mode [13]. The transfer mode occurs during normal waking and is characterized by a constant firing rate. In this mode, thalamic cells faithfully relay afferent signals to the cortex. The oscillatory mode occurs during drowsiness and slow wave sleep [13]. In this mode, thalamic cells fire in high-frequency bursts of action potentials preceded by a prolonged decrease in firing rate.

The mechanisms associated with the constant firing rate of thalamic neurons observed during waking and the bursting observed during sleep have recently been clarified [14]. The transfer mode occurs when the membrane of a thalamocortical cell is held depolarized above resting membrane potential but below threshold. The bursting associated with the oscillatory mode occurs during prolonged hyperpolarization which enables a calcium conductance or calcium spike [15]. During calcium spikes the cell fires a series of action potentials at high frequency – a calcium spike-associated burst [15, 16]. Calcium spike-associated bursts are characterized by a short initial interspike interval (ISI) followed by ISIs that become progressively longer throughout the burst [17, 18].

Intraburst ISI structure can be studied by segregating bursts by the number of ISIs occurring in each burst. The average duration of ISIs is then determined as a function of the ordinal of the ISI within bursts of different lengths. The average duration of an ISI is then plotted as a function of the ordinal number of the ISI [19]. By this method, a single cell undergoing calcium spike-associated bursting should show positive slopes for all bursts, regardless of the number of action potentials per burst.

In the ventrolateral nucleus of naturally sleeping cats bursting is known to be associated with calcium spikes and is characterized by positive slopes and short intraburst ISIs -2.6 ± 0.8 ms ($\overline{x} \pm SD$) [18]. The structure of these bursts is very similar across different nuclei and species [14, 18]. In a sleeping patient, positive slopes were found for all bursts regardless of numbers of spikes per burst (3 cells). The duration of intraburst ISIs in these bursts was 4.6 ± 1.1 ms [Lenz et al., unpubl. observations]. Although the number of cells in sleeping humans is very small, the ISI pattern of these bursts is very similar to that seen in the sleeping cat [Steriade, personal commun.].

In 3 patients with central pain following spinal cord transection, positive slopes were found for all bursts in 20 of 25 cells located in the region of ventrocaudal thalamus representing the part of the body where the patient experiences pain [19]. The mean intraburst ISI duration was 2.5 ± 1.0 ms. These results demonstrate that calcium spike-associated bursting can also occur in waking patients with some pathologic conditions.

Studies of the intraburst ISI structure of thalamic bursts in parkinsonian patients suggest that calcium spike-associated bursting does not fully explain tremor-related activity [Lenz et al., unpubl. observations]. In recordings from 25 cells in presumed Vim and Vop of parkinsonian patients, the average duration of intraburst ISIs was 16 ± 12 ms. Positive slopes were found for one cell of 25 showing significant correlation between tremor related activity and EMG activity. For this cell, the average duration of intraburst ISIs was 17 ± 11 ms. The differences in intraburst ISI structure and ISI duration suggest that tremor related activity is different from the bursting seen in sleeping cats and humans.

Basal Ganglia Oscillators Potentially Involved in Tremor

Ventralis oralis anterior and Vop are connected to the basal ganglia through a circuit that takes origin from pre- and post-central sensorimotor cortex and involves portions of the putamen, globus pallidus and subthalamic nucleus. The main output of the basal ganglia is the inhibitory (GABAergic) connection from the internal segment of the globus pallidus (GPi) to Vop [20–22], termed VLo in monkeys [23]. Studies of GPi in monkeys made parkinsonian by administration of MPTP (1-methyl-4-phenyl-1,2,3,6-tetrahydropyridine) demonstrate increased tonic activity and abnormal bursting activity related to tremor [24, 25]. In guinea pig GP, corresponding to the external segment of GP in primates, a population of cells has a natural tendency to oscillate in the 4–6 Hz range when depolarized from a hyperpolarized membrane potential [26]. Similar cells in primates might result in oscillations reflected in thalamic tremor-related activity. The suggestion that a central oscillator is located in basal ganglia is also supported by the finding that lesions of GPi are effective in relieving parkinsonian tremor [27, 28].

Since efferents from GPi inhibit Vop, the increase in tonic activity in GPi might produce hyperpolarization of thalamocortical cells and so generate thalamic calcium spike-associated bursting. In this formulation, thalamic tremor-related activity should show the calcium spike-associated burst pattern [5, 6]. However, bursts recorded in thalamus of parkinsonian patients are much different than those associated with calcium spikes (see above). These results suggest that thalamic tremor-related activity may arise due to transmission of bursting activity from GPi to cells in Vop which are in the transfer mode, i.e. slightly depolarized.

Peripheral Hypothesis

The Effects of Peripheral Inputs upon Tremor

Studies of tremor in parkinsonian patients and primate models of parkinsonism can be interpreted to suggest that tremor occurs in the absence of peripheral inputs. In the monkey model of rest tremor produced by a lesion of the ventromedial midbrain tegmentum, tremor persists following dorsal root section [51]. Furthermore, dorsal root section in a parkinsonian patient did not abolish the tremor although it did alter the '... amplitude, rhythm and rate' of tremor. This latter result may suggest that peripheral inputs are not essential but do play a modulatory role in the generation of tremor [29].

The influence of peripheral inputs on tremor characteristics may be assessed by resetting studies, which measure the extent to which peripheral stimuli reset or alter tremor. Electrical stimulation of peripheral nerves can alter the frequency, amplitude and phase of tremor [30]. In addition, sinusoidal driving of the joints during tremor evokes EMG activity that is temporally locked to the stretch of the muscle [31]. Finally, short perturbations of the tremulous joint may alter the phase of tremor [32 cf. 3].

While resetting studies suggest that peripheral inputs play a modulatory role in parkinsonian tremor, they must be interpreted cautiously. The interpretation of resetting studies is complicated by the observation that a change in phase can follow muscle contraction and can be related to the silent period following both the M response and the H response [30]. Furthermore, since the EMG and mechanical components of tremor can be varied independently by changing the mechanical parameters of the system [1, 33], changes in phase produced by peripheral stimuli might result from mechanical properties of the system in addition to physiologic activity.

Evidence that Peripheral Inputs Play a Role in Human Thalamic Tremor-Related Activity

The possibility that sensory feedback influences human thalamic tremor-related activity has been assessed by comparing the activity of cells in presumed Vim and Vop with sensory inputs to that of cells without sensory input. Cells with activity related to active movement are classified into those that are also activated in response to somatosensory stimulation (combined cells), and those that are not (voluntary cells) [34–37]. Combined cells are activated in advance of EMG activity during active movement and so can be distinguished from sensory cells that respond only to somatosensory stimulation [34].

Since movement leads to somatosensory input that is transmitted to the thalamus after a conduction delay, tremor-related activity of sensory cells might be expected to lag behind tremor. As predicted, the activity of the majority of thalamic sensory cells lagged tremor in parkinsonian patients. The activity of a majority of combined and voluntary cells was correlated with and led tremor. This suggests that the tremor-related activity of combined cells is related to peripheral inputs in a way which is different from that of sensory cells in Vc. Although the fact that thalamic activity leads tremor does not prove that thalamic activity causes tremor, the similarities between the tremor-related activity of combined and voluntary cell types may suggest that both are involved in the generation of tremor.

Peripheral mechanisms may play a role in the tremor-related activity of voluntary as well as combined cells. Systems analysis techniques demonstrate evidence of feedback mechanisms in the transfer function linking tremor with thalamic tremor-related activity [38]. More than 90% of cells in presumed Vim and Vop without a response to somatosensory stimulation [39] showed evidence of a feedback mechanism. These cells may have somatosensory inputs from a wide somatotopic area, making detection of the sensory response difficult (see below). Taken together, the results reviewed in this section suggest that somatosensory mechanisms may have a role in the generation of thalamic tremor-related activity and tremor.

CNS Pathways through which Peripheral Inputs Might Influence Tremor-Related Activity

Short Latency Somatosensory Inputs to Motor Cortex via Vim. One hypothesis which seeks to explain the role of peripheral input in parkinsonian symptoms is the long loop reflex hypothesis. Long loop reflex arcs are postulated to traverse peripheral nerves, dorsal column nuclei, thalamic nuclei, motor cortex, and, finally, spinal motor neurons in much the same way as segmental stretch reflexes traverse the spinal cord [40]. Recent studies have demonstrated short latency inputs to monkey VPLo, corresponding to human Vim [23]. VPLo primarily projects to motor cortex [37], where spike triggered averaging studies demonstrate that responses of neurons to peripheral inputs are appropriately timed for involvement of these neurons in long latency reflex activity [41].

Therefore, transmission of afferent input through this long loop reflex arc may contribute to long latency stretch reflex activity [42–44]. Simulation studies have shown that transmission of afferent activity through long loop reflex arcs, which have become unstable as a result of increased gain, is theoretically capable of producing parkinsonian tremor [45].

The long loop hypothesis of tremor is supported by studies showing increased gain of long latency reflex activity in parkinsonian patients [46–49], tending to make this feedback circuit unstable [45]. Additionally, studies of neuronal activity along the proposed long loop reflex pathway demonstrate increased responses to peripheral inputs as would be predicted by this mechanism. For example, neurons in precentral cortex of phenothiazine intoxicated monkeys demonstrate increased responses to peripheral stimulation. Additionally, the phase of cortical tremor related activity is altered by perturbations of the tremulous joint [50]. However, the fact that motor cortical bursting activity persists following curarization may suggest that this activity is not solely generated by peripheral inputs [4, 51].

Somatosensory Inputs to Motor Cortex from the Basal Ganglia 'Motor' Circuit via Vop. Cells in the basal ganglia 'motor' circuit demonstrate increased responses to peripheral inputs [24, 25]. This finding raises the possibility that the increased precentral cortical responses in parkinsonian tremor models may occur by transmission of basal ganglia output via Vop to the cortex. Neurons in GPi demonstrate responses to peripheral stimulation that are increased in both magnitude and duration in MPTP-treated monkeys [24, 25]. These neurons project to monkey VLo, corresponding to human Vop [52], where cells in MPTP-treated monkeys demonstrate responses to somatosensory stimuli that are much more frequent and less specific [35]. Neurons in VLo project to the 'hand representation' of primary motor cortex [53]. In this way, activity in the basal ganglia 'motor' circuit might explain the changes in motor cortical responses to peripheral input (see above).

Conclusions

In summary, the evidence suggests that the mechanism linking the thalamus to parkinsonian tremor involves a central oscillator. Human studies suggest that the calcium spike-associated oscillator may not completely explain thalamic tremor-related activity. It is possible that other thalamic oscillators, unexplored at present, may be involved. However, tremor-related activity might also be explained by transmission through the thalamus of activity generated by a central oscillator located elsewhere – perhaps in the basal ganglia.

In addition, peripheral inputs seem to influence thalamic tremor-related activity that may be involved in the generation of tremor. This may occur through at least two mechanisms – a short latency direct pathway to motor cortex or an indirect pathway via the basal ganglia. This sensory input may modulate the activity of the central oscillator and significantly influence the characteristics of parkinsonian tremor.

Acknowledgement

Some of the studies described in this paper were supported by grants from the National Institutes of Health to F.A.L. (K08-NS01384, R29-28598), J.L.V. (K08-NS01328) and M.R.D. (P50-NS20471). We wish to thank Mrs. Beth Norris who typed this manuscript.

References

1 Elble RJ, Koller W: Tremor. Baltimore, Johns Hopkins University Press, 1990.
2 Marsden CD: Origins of normal and pathological tremor; in Findley LJ, Capildeo R (eds): Movement Disorders: Tremor. London, Macmillan Press, 1984, pp 37–85.
3 Stein RB, Lee RG: Tremor and clonus; in Brooks VB (ed): Handbook of Physiology. Motor Control. Bethesda, American Physiological Society, 1981, pp 325–343.
4 Lamarre Y, Joffroy AJ: Experimental tremor in monkey: Activity of thalamic and precentral cortical neurons in the absence of peripheral feedback. Adv Neurol 1979;24:109–122.
5 Parc D, Curro Dossi R, Steriade M: Neuronal basis of the parkinsonian resting tremor: A hypothesis and its implications for treatment. Neuroscience 1990;35: 217–226.
6 Buzsaki G, Smith A, Berger S, et al: Petit mal epilepsy and parkinsonian tremor: Hypothesis of a common pacemaker. Neuroscience 1990;36:1–14.
7 Hassler R: Anatomy of the thalamus; in Schaltenbrand G, Bailey P (eds): Introduction to Stereotaxis with an Atlas of the Human Brain. Stuttgart, Thieme, 1959, pp 230–290.
8 Hirai T, Jones EG: Distribution of tachykinin- and enkephalin-immunoreactive fibers in the human thalamus. Brain Res Rev 1989;14:35–52.
9 Jones EG: The Thalamus. New York, Plenum Press, 1985.
10 Lenz FA, Tasker RR, Kwan HC, et al: Single unit analysis of the human ventral thalamic nuclear group: Correlation of thalamic 'tremor cells' with the 3–6 Hz component of parkinsonian tremor. J Neurosci 1988;8:754–764.
11 Lenz FA, Tasker RR, Kwan HC, et al: Single unit analysis of the ventral tier of lateral thalamic nuclei in patients with parkinsonian tremor. Soc Neurosci Abstr 1985;11:1164.
12 Tasker RR, Siqueira J, Hawrylyshyn PA, et al: What happened to VIM thalamotomy for Parkinson's disease? Appl Neurophysiol 1983;46:68–83.
13 Steriade M, Deschenes M: The thalamus as a neuronal oscillator. Brain Res Rev 1984;8:1–63.
14 Steriade M, Jones EG, Llinas RR: Thalamic Oscillations and Signaling. New York, Wiley, 1990.
15 Jahnsen H, Lllinas R: Ionic basic for the electroresponsiveness and oscillatory properties of guinea-pig thalamic neurons in vitro. J Physiol 1984;349:247–349.
16 Roy JP, Clercq M, Steriade M, et al: Electrophysiology of neurons of lateral thalamic nuclei in cat: mechanisms of long-lasting hyperpolarizations. J Neurophysiol 1984;51:1220–1235.
17 Deschenes M, Paradis M, Roy JP, et al: Electrophysiology of neurons of lateral thalamic nuclei in cat: resting properties and burst discharges. J Neurophysiol 1984;51:1196–1219.
18 Domich L, Oakson G, Steriade M: Thalamic burst patterns in the naturally sleeping cat: A comparison between cortically-projecting and reticularis neurones. J Physiol 1986;379:429–449.
19 Lenz FA, Kwan HC, Dostrovsky JO, et al: Characteristics of the bursting pattern of action potentials that occur in the thalamus of patients with central pain. Brain Res 1989;496:357–360.

20 Alexander GE, DeLong MR, Strick PL: Parallel organization of functionally segregated circuits linking basal ganglia and cortex. Annu Rev Neurosci 1986;9:357–381.
21 Alexander GE, Crutcher MD: Functional architecture of basal ganglia circuits: neural substrates of parallel processing. Trends Neurosci 1990;13:266–271.
22 DeLong MR: Primate models of movement disorders of basal ganglia origin. Trends Neurosci 1990;13:281–285.
23 Olszewski J: The Thalamus of *Macaca mulatta.* Basel, Karger, 1952.
24 Miller WC, DeLong MR: Parkinsonian symptomatology: Anatomical and physiological analysis. Ann NY Acad Sci 1988;515:287–302.
25 Filion M, Tremblay L, Bedard PJ: Abnormal influences of passive limb movement on the activity of globus pallidus neurons in parkinsonian monkeys. Brain Res 1988;444:165–176.
26 Nambu A, Llinas R: Electrophysiology of the globus pallidus neurons: An in vitro study in guinea pig brain slices. Soc Neurosci Abstr 1990;16:428.
27 Laitinen LV, Hariz MI: Pallidal surgery abolishes parkinsonian symptoms. Mov Disord 1990;5:82.
28 Svennilson E, Torvik A, Lowe R, et al: Treatment of parkinsonism by stereotactic thermolesions in the pallidal region. Acta Psychiatr Neurol Scand 1960;35:358–377.
29 Pollack LJ, Davis L: Muscle tone in parkinsonian states. Arch Neurol Psychiatry 1930;23:303–319.
30 Renou G, Rondot P, Bathien N: Influence of peripheral stimulation on the silent period between bursts of parkinsonian tremor; in Desmedt JE (ed): New Developments in Electromyography and Clinical Neurophysiology. Karger, Basel, 1973, pp 635–640.
31 Rack PMH, Ross HF: The role of reflexes in the resting tremor of Parkinson's disease. Brain 1986;109:115–141.
32 Teravainen H, Evarts E, Calne D: Effects of kinesthetic inputs on parkinsonian tremor. Adv Neurol 1979;24:161–173.
33 Rack PMH: Mechanical and reflex factors in human tremor, in Desmedt JE (ed): Physiological Tremor, Pathological Tremor and Clonus. Basel, Karger, 1973, pp 17–28.
34 Lenz FA, Kwan H, Dostrovsky JO, et al: Single unit analysis of the human ventral thalamic nuclear group: Activity correlated with movement. Brain 1990;113:1795–1821.
35 Vitek JL, Ashe J, De Long MR, et al: Altered Somatosensory response properties of neurons in the 'motor' thalamus of MPTP treated parkinsonian monkeys. Soc Neurosci Abstr 1990;16:425.
36 Ashe J, Vitek JL, DeLong MR, et al: Evidence for somatotopic organization within thalamic nucleus VLo (ventralis lateralis pars oralis). Soc Neurosci Abstr 1990;16:425.
37 Vitek JL, Ashe J, DeLong MR, et al: Organization of primate ventrolateral thalamus: Neuronal relations to active and passive limb movements. Soc Neurosci Abstr 1989;15:287.
38 Schnider SM, Kwong RH, Lenz FA, et al: Detection of feedback in the central nervous system using system identification techniques. Biol Cybern 1989;60:203–212.

39 Lenz FA, Dostrovsky JO, Tasker RR, et al: Single-unit analysis of the human ventral thalamic nuclear group: Somatosensory responses. J Neurophysiol 1988;59: 299–316.
40 Desmedt JE: Progress in Clinical Neurophysiology. Cerebral Motor Control in Man: Long Loop Mechanisms. Basel, Karger, 1978.
41 Cheney PD, Fetz EE: Corticoneuronal cells contribute to long-latency stretch reflexes in the rhesus monkey. J Physiol 1984;349:249–272.
42 Lenz FA, Tatton WG, Tasker RR: Electromyographic response to displacement of different forelimb joints in the squirrel monkey. J Neurosci 1983;3:783–794.
43 Lenz FA, Tatton WG, Tasker RR: The effect of cortical lesions on the electromyographic response to joint displacement in the squirrel monkey forelimb. J Neurosci 1983;3:795–805.
44 Marsden CD, Merton PA, Morton HB: Latency measurements compatible with a cortical pathway for the stretch reflex in man. J Physiol 1973;230:58–59.
45 Stein RB, Oguztoreli MN: Tremor and other oscillations in neuromuscular systems. Biol Cybern 1976;22:147–157.
46 Tatton WG, Lee RG: Evidence for abnormal long-loop reflexes in rigid parkinsonian patients. Brain Res 1975;100:671–676.
47 Chan CWY, Kearney RE, Jones G Melvill: Tibialis anterior response to sudden ankle displacement in normal and parkinsonian subjects. Brain Res 1979;173:303–314.
48 Rothwell JC, Obeso JA, Traub MM, et al: The behavior of long-latency stretch reflex in patients with Parkinson's disease. J Neurol Neurosurg Psychiatry 1983;46: 35–44.
49 Struppler F, Lehmann-Horn F, Klein W, et al: Effect of stereoencephalotomy on long-latency EMG responses and motor control of arm movements in Parkinson's syndrome. Adv Neurol 1984;40:437–445.
50 Tatton WG, Bawa P, Bruce IC: Altered motor cortical activity in extrapyramidal rigidity. Adv Neurol 1979;24:141–160.
51 Ohye C, Bouchard R, Larochelle L, et al: Effect of dorsal rhizotomy on postural tremor in the monkey. Exp Brain Res 1970;10:140–150.
52 Hirai T, Jones EG: A new parcellation of the human thalamus on the basis of histochemical staining. Brain Res Rev 1989;14:1–34.
53 Holsapple JW, Preston JB, Strick PL: Origin of thalamic inputs to the 'hand'. Representation in the primary motor cortex. Soc Neurosci Abstr 1990;16:425.

F.A. Lenz, MD, Department of Neurosurgery, Meyer Building 7-113,
Johns Hopkins Hospital, 600 North Wolfe Street, Baltimore, MD 21205 (USA)

Proceedings of the 2nd International Workshop on Microphysiological Recordings during Stereotactic Neurosurgery: Motor Thalamus, October 1–2, 1989, Nikko, Japan
Stereotact Funct Neurosurg 1993;60:104–120

Action of the Cerebello-Thalamo-Cortical Projection upon Visually Initiated Reaction-Time Hand Movements in the Monkey

Kazuo Sasaki, Hisae Gemba

Department of Integrative Brain Science, Faculty of Medicine, Kyoto University, Kyoto, Japan

Key Words. Cerebral cortex · Thalamo-cortical response · Motor learning · Field potential · Cerebellum · Compensation

Abstract. Electrophysiological characterization of thalamo-cortical projections and cerebello-thalamo-cortical pathways was shown by acute experiments in which laminar field potential analysis of responses evoked in the cortex by stimulation of thalamic and cerebellar nuclei was performed in anesthetized monkeys. Based on the results, dynamic activities of cerebro-cerebellar interconnections on voluntary movements were recorded with electrodes chronically implanted in various cortical areas in unanesthetized monkeys and were correlated with their behaviours. Cortical field potentials change in learning processes of visually initiated reaction-time hand movement and in compensating processes after cerebellar hemispherectomy.

Thalamo-Cortical Projection as Studied by Laminar Field Potential Analysis in the Cortex

Our laminar field potential analysis of responses evoked in the cortex by stimulation of thalamic nuclei was made first in cats [1, 2] and then in monkeys [3], following many previous morphological and physiological investigations [4, 5]. In cats, the analysis suggested the exis-

1011–6125/93/0603–0104 $ 2.75/0

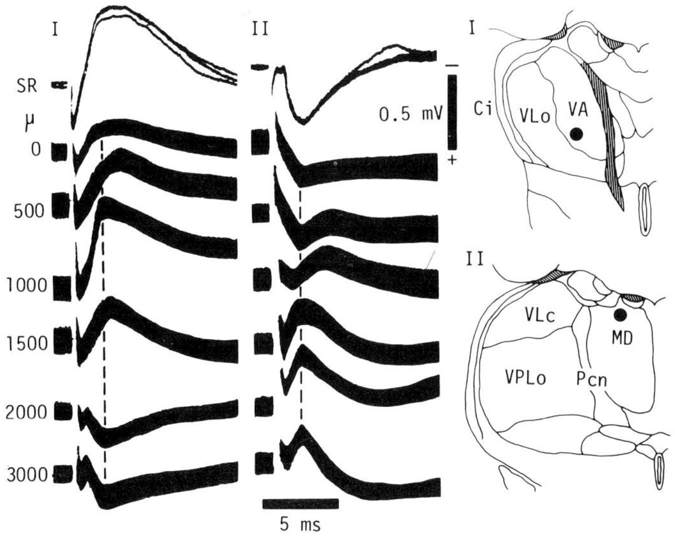

Fig. 1. Superficial (I) and deep (II) thalamo-cortical (T-C) responses recorded at 0–3,000 μm depths of the same microelectrode track in the premotor cortex of a monkey. Stimulation (0.5 ms duration, 1 mA strength, delivered at a 2-second interval) was given to the VA (I) and MD (II) thalamic nucleus as marked by filled circles in the right diagrams of the frontal section. Nomenclature of the thalamic nuclei was according to Olszewski. SR row was taken by a silver ball electrode placed near the microelectrode track on the cortical surface, and other rows were by a glass microelectrode filled with 2 *M* NaCl solution and inserted at various depths (indicated in μm to the left). Peaks of the reversed potentials are marked by vertical broken lines. About 10 sweeps were superimposed. 0.5 mV calibration for the microelectrode records. 5 ms time scale for all records.

tence of two different kinds of thalamo-cortical (T-C) projections, i.e. superficial and deep T-C ones, of which the stimulation elicited entirely different laminar field potentials in the cortex, called respectively superficial and deep T-C responses [1]. The same kind of study was then performed in monkeys and the essentially same characterization of thalamo-cortical projections as in cats could be found [3, 6]. Examples of the responses in monkeys are shown in figures 1 and 2.

Recording with a microelectrode inserted at different depths in a locus in the premotor cortex (area 6) revealed superficial (I) and deep (II) T-C responses on stimulation of the VA (I) and MD (II) thalamic

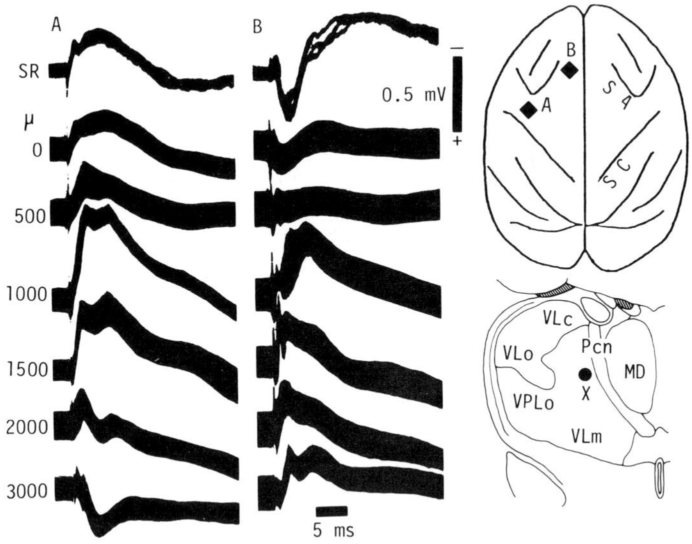

Fig. 2. Stimulation (0.5 ms duration, 1 mA strength, delivered at 2 s interval) of the X nucleus (VL) induced, respectively, a superficial T-C response in the forelimb motor cortex (A) and a deep T-C response in the premotor cortex (B) in a monkey. Other indications are the same as in figure 1.

nucleus of a monkey (fig. 1). The VA stimulation induced surface-negative, depth-positive (s-N, d-P) field potentials, which reversed their polarity between 1,500 and 2,000 μm from the cortical surface, whereas the MD stimulation elicited s-P, d-N potentials, of which the polarity turned at around 500 μm depth. This indicates that different thalamic nuclei project upon the same cortical locus with the different T-C projections. Figure 2 shows another example which presents that stimulation of a thalamic locus produces a superficial T-C response in the forelimb area of the motor cortex and a deep T-C response in the premotor cortex. Such studies suggest that every cortical response due to T-C inputs is a simple T-C response by either of the two T-C projections or a spatial and/or temporal admixture of both responses [1].

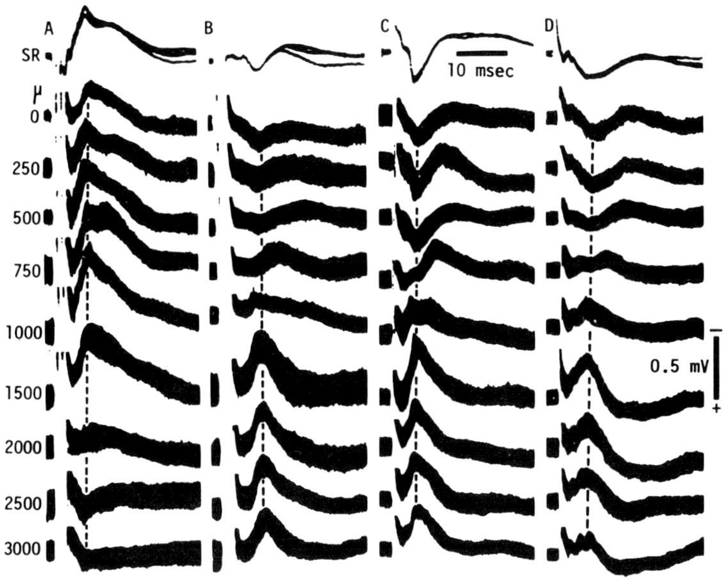

Fig. 3. Laminar field potentials in the motor cortex in response to stimulation of the cerebellar lateral nucleus (A), the cerebellar medial nucleus (B), the ipsilateral premotor cortex (C), and the contralateral motor cortex (D), respectively. They were all recorded in the same microelectrode track. Depths from the cortical surface are given to the left in μm. SR indicates the surface potentials recorded with a silver ball electrode placed near the microelectrode track. 0.5 mV microelectrode records. 10 ms for all records. Vertical broken lines connect the peaks of reversed potentials in respective responses. From Sasaki et al. [6].

The electrophysiological characterization of T-C projections as proposed [1–3, 6] have been well supported by later morphological investigations [7–11].

Cerebro-Cerebellar Interconnection

Stimulation of cerebellar nuclei induced superficial or deep T-C responses in the motor (area 4), premotor (area 6) and parietal association (area 5) cortices [3], as well as the frontal association cortex (area 9) [12]. Stimulation of the medial nucleus elicits deep T-C responses in

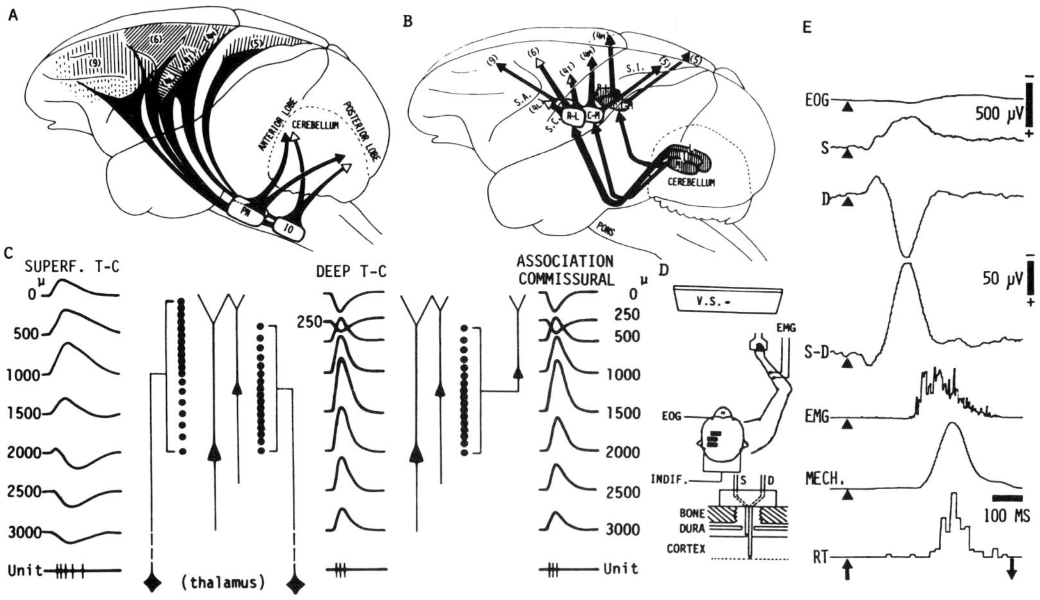

Fig. 4A, B. Diagrams of cerebro-cerebellar interconnections in monkeys. Numbers indicate the different cortical areas after Brodmann. Area 4 is divided into lateral (4L), intermediate (4I) and medial (4M) parts. PN = Pontine nuclei; IO = inferior olive; S.A. = arcuate sulcus; S.C. = central sulcus; S.I. = intraparietal sulcus; M, I, L = medial, interpositus, lateral nuclei of the cerebellum; R-L, C-M = two nuclear complexes of the thalamus. **C** Diagram of laminar field potentials in the cortex by the two thalamo-cortical (superficial and deep T-C) and the cortico-cortical (association or commissural) inputs. Numbers indicate the depth from the cortical surface in μm. Unit = Schematic pattern of firing of cortical pyramidal neurone. The presumed excitatory synaptic terminals on apical dendrites of cortical pyramidal neurones in layers III and V are shown diagrammatically by dots for the three afferent inputs. Laminar field potentials are attributed to electrical dipoles generated in pyramidal neurones by the EPSPs. **D** Diagram of the methods of chronic experiments with monkeys as described in the methods of the text. In the lower part, electrodes placed on the cortical surface (S) and in 2.0–3.0 mm depth (D) through the bone and dura are illustrated. **E** Examples of EOG, cortical potentials (S, D, S-D), EMG, mechanogram of lever movement (Mech.) and reaction time histogram (RT) are presented as explained in the text. 500 μV for EOG and 50 μV for cortical potentials. 100 ms for all traces. Modified from Sasaki [15].

a relatively medial part of area 4 (mainly hindlimb motor area) and area 5 on both contra- and ipsilateral sides. Stimulation of the interpositus nucleus evokes superficial T-C responses in an intermediate part of area 4 (truncal and proximal limb motor area) and area 6 on the contralateral side. Stimulation of the lateral nucleus produces superficial T-C responses in a relatively lateral part of area 4 (forelimb motor area) and area 6 on the contralateral side. In addition to it, lateral nucleus stimulation sets up deep T-C responses in a dorsal part of area 9 and its continuation to the rostral partof area 6 [12]. Figure 3 shows examples of superficial T-C responses by lateral nucleus stimulation (A), deep T-C responses by medial nucleus stimulation (B) and cortico-cortical (C-C) responses by stimulation of the ipsilateral premotor cortex (C) and by that of the contralateral motor cortex (D), being recorded from one and the same microelectrode track in the motor cortex [6].

These T-C and C-C responses are summarized as half-schematical laminar field potentials, and assumed synaptic terminals on cortical pyramidal neurons in layers III and V are drawn in figure 4c. In figure 4b, the cerebello-thalamo-cortical projections are illustrated in a simplified schema. Cortico-cerebellar projections were studied in cats [13] and monkeys [14], and those of monkeys are shown in figure 4a. In brief, the forelimb motor area (4L), premotor area (6) and prefrontal area (9) project mainly onto the neocerebellum (posterior lobe, lateral part or hemispherical part of the cerebellum) via the pontine nuclei and inferior olive. The hindlimb motor area (4M) and the parietal association area (5) go mainly to the paleocerebellum (anterior lobe, intermediate and medial part of the cerebellum). The intermediate motor area (4I) gives intermediate projections between those of 4L and 4M to the cerebellum.

These features of cerebro-cerebellar interconnections in monkeys inspired us to investigate cerebro-cerebellar interactions for organization and control of voluntary hand movements, since it was postulated that the prefrontal and premotor projection onto the neocerebellum and the neocerebellar projection in turn onto the forelimb motor cortex must be an essential neuronal circuit for initiation of voluntary hand movement [15, cf. 16, 17]. It has been especially advantageous for us to study the conditioned hand movement in monkeys, as the forelimb motor area receives mainly and almost exclusively the neocerebellar output via superficial T-C projections.

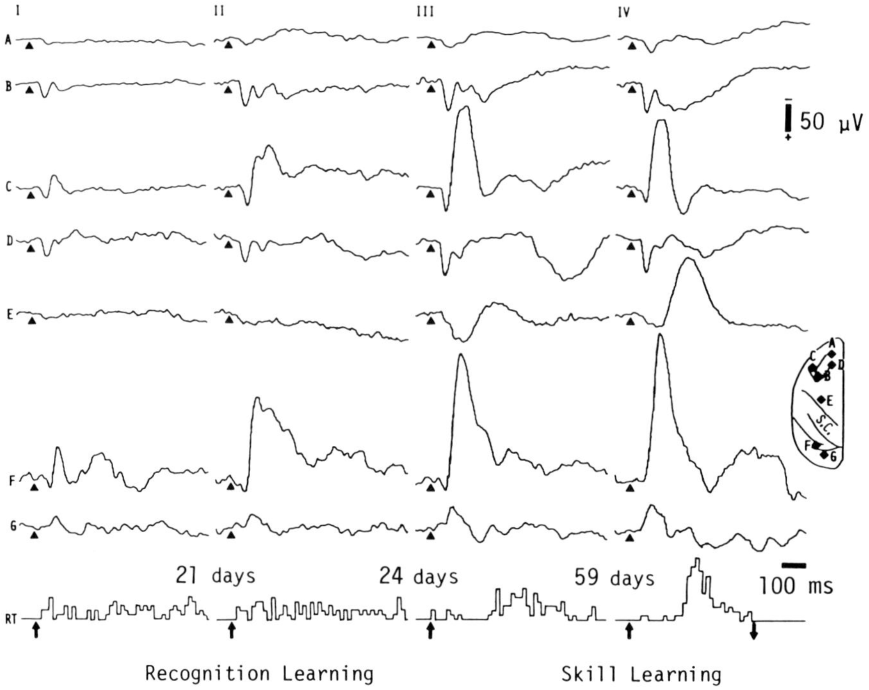

Fig. 5. Premovement S-D potentials in seven cortical loci on the left hemisphere of a monkey learning the reaction-time movement of the right hand. Columns I-IV present four sessions at different stages. I was taken in the second session, and II, III and IV were taken, respectively, 21, 24 and 59 days after session I. Potentials were averaged 100 times from every session for respective cortical loci indicated by alphabetical symbols in the inset diagram and each row of records. The stimulus was given for 900 ms at stage I–III but 510 ms at IV. Only the movements which occurred during the light stimulus were counted in RT histograms and averaged potentials (the later part of 900 ms is curtailed in columns I–III). They were aligned by the stimulus onset pulse as indicated by triangle and upward arrow, the downward arrow showing the end of 510 ms stimulus. 50 μV for all potentials and 100 ms for all traces. Modified from Sasaki and Gemba [19].

Dynamic Activities of Cerebro-Cerebellar Interconnections in Voluntary Movements

Methods

Adult monkeys *(Macaca fuscata)* were trained to lift a lever with wrist extension in response to a light stimulus. The stimulus lasted for about 500 ms and was delivered at random time intervals of 2.5–6.0 s. The monkey had to move the hand within the duration of the visual stimulus given in front of the monkey by a diode emitting green light (V.S. in fig. 4d). At first the monkey moved the hand in his own time without regard to the light stimulus but gradually learned to perform the reaction-time movement (fig. 5).

Electrodes for recording cortical field potentials consist of silver needles (about 250 μm in diameter) insulated except for their pointed tips. A pair of them were placed, respectively, on the surface and at 2.0–3.0 mm depth in the cerebral cortex and fixed to the bone by dental cement (fig. 4D, lower part). Usually 15–20 pairs of such electrodes were implanted in each hemisphere and served for recording for more than several months. Cortical field potentials were recorded against indifferent electrodes buried in the bone behind the ear on both sides (Indif., fig. 4D), amplified through 2.0-second time constant amplifiers and recorded on magnetic tapes, together with pulses of stimulus onset and movement onset etc. An electro-oculogram (EOG) led from the rostrolateral edge of the frontal bone was monitored. Examples are shown in figure 4E of EOG, surface (S), depth (D), surface minus depth (S-D) potentials from the forelimb motor cortex contralateral to the moving hand in a well-trained monkey, being averaged 100 times by the stimulus onset pulse (triangle and upward arrow). Electromyogram (EMG) recorded bipolarly from the skin over wrist extensor muscles was rectified and likewise averaged, and the lever movement was converted to electrical signal and aligned 100 times (Mech.). Reaction times of the 100 movements are given in a histogram of 16-ms bins (RT) where the onset and end of the stimulus are indicated by upward and downward arrows.

Contribution of each cortical area to the conditioned movement and functional significance of cortical potentials on the movement were investigated by cooling temporarily each area [18]. For local cooling, metal chambers, of which the undersides were shaped so as to cover the respective cortical areas to be cooled, were placed on several areas in each hemisphere and fixed to the bone by dental cement. Every chamber had input and output pipes which were connected to a pump for perfusing warm (38–39 °C) or cold (about 1 °C) water. The silver needle electrodes were set under the chamber to record cortical field potentials in the control and cooling states.

In some experiments, the cerebellar hemisphere ipsilateral to the operant hand was resected, after the monkey had been well trained with the reaction-time hand movement, in order to observe changes of the movement and cortical field potentials due to the operation. The cerebellar hemispherectomy usually included both the lateral and interpositus nuclei. The extent of the operation was checked histologically after electrophysiological experiments had lasted for several months. The sites of recording electrodes in the cortex were also examined morphologically after the experiments.

Development and Change of Cortical Field Potentials during Learning Processes of Conditioned Hand Movement

Field potentials in various cortical areas were successively measured for several months in which untaught monkeys gradually learned the reaction-time hand movement in response to the light stimulus and reached the well-established state [19]. Figure 5 presents examples of seven cortical loci (A-G) contralateral to the moving hand in one and the same monkey. As seen in the reaction time histogram (RT), the monkey initially lifted the lever at its self pace without regard to the light stimulus (900 ms duration starting at the upward arrow, the end part being curtailed). Only the movements which occurred incidentally during the light stimulus were sampled in the RT histogram. Alignment of cortical field potentials (surface minus depth potentials in A-G rows) by the onset pulse of stimulus revealed some significant responses in the prefrontal (A-C), premotor (D), prestriate (F) and striate (G) cortices even at this unlearned stage (column I). These responses gradually increased in size on each day of training (column II) until stage III when the monkey started to move the hand in response to the light stimulus (column III). Reaction times were longer than stage IV (column IV) and many trials occurred out of the stimulus duration. At this stage, s-P, d-N potentials appeared in the forelimb motor cortex (E row) at a latency of about 50 ms.

After stage III, repeated trainings hardly changed the potentials in the association and premotor cortices but added gradually the s-N, d-P potential in the forelimb motor cortex at a latency of about 120 ms in parallel with faster and less variable reaction times, i.e. better timing of the movement (column IV, E and RT rows). The s-N, d-P potential in the forelimb motor cortex (see also fig. 4E) can be attributed to the response elicited by the volley through the neocerebellum and the thala-

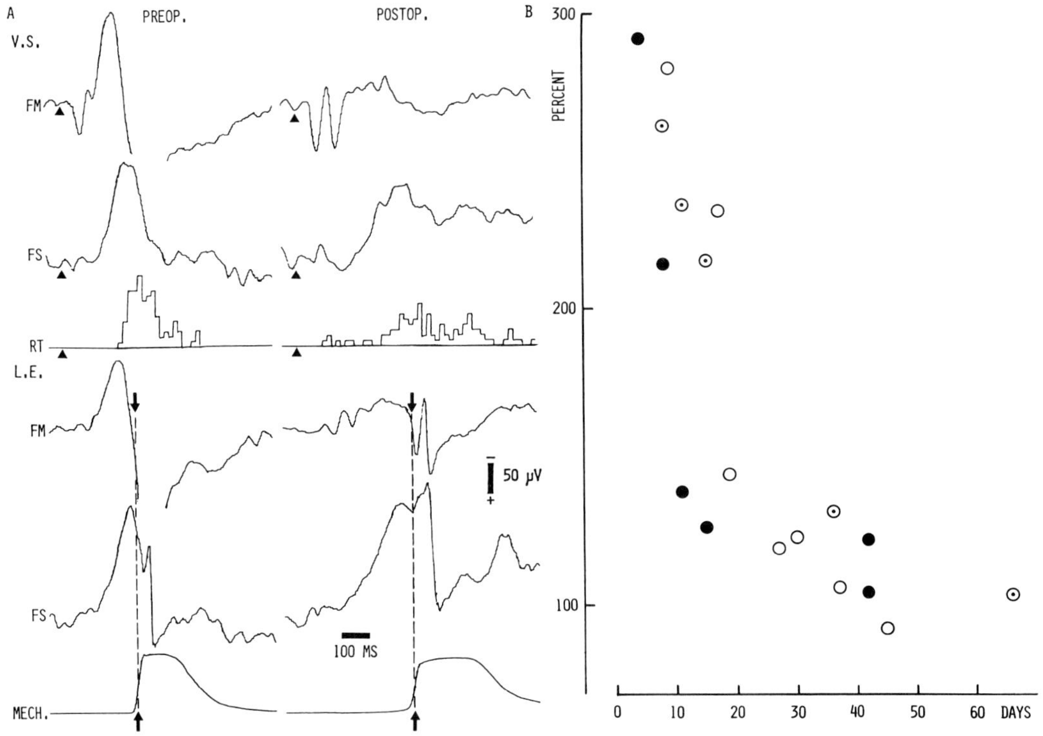

Fig. 6. A Field potentials (S-D) from the forelimb motor (FM) and somatosensory (FS) cortices associated with visually initiated hand movements before and after cerebellar hemispherectomy in a monkey. The same data were aligned 100 times by the stimulus onset (triangle) (upper half, VS) and the movement onset (arrows with broken line) (lower half, LE) pulses, respectively. The VS averages are accompanied with reaction time histograms (RT) and the LE averages with mechanograms (Mech.). 50 µV for all cortical potentials and 100 ms for all traces. **B** Enhancement of the premovement component of the somatosensory potentials after cerebellar hemispherectomy is plotted against days after the operation (abscissa). The premovement area of the S-D potential is plotted on the ordinate as a percentage of the preoperative value. The three symbols indicate data from three different monkeys. Modified from Sasaki and Gemba [24].

mus, which had been supported by several sorts of experiments, as partly exemplified later [19, 20]. Thus, it is considered that the gradual recruitment of cerebro-cerebellar interaction is closely correlated with attaining fast and fixed reaction times of movements. Quick and appropriate timing is undoubtedly one of the most important factors of skilled intended movements, and the process from stage III to IV may be called 'skill learning', in contrast to the process from stage I to III, which can be called 'recognition learning' in associating the visual stimulus with the movement [19, 21].

The idea that the recruitment of cerebro-cerebellar interaction is indispensable to skill learning was supported also by ablation experiment of the cerebellar hemisphere in well-trained monkeys [20] and in untaught monkeys [19]. Ablation of the cerebellar hemisphere in well-trained monkeys cancelled the skill learning and degraded the movement at stage IV to stage III (fig. 6). The ablation in untaught monkeys made to promote the learning processes only until stage III and the monkeys never reached stage IV [19].

It would be worthwhile to mention here that degradation of the reaction-time movement from stage III to I or II, namely cancellation of the recognition learning, was partly made by local cooling of the premotor cortex in both cerebral hemispheres [22].

Compensation after Localized Ablation or Cooling of the Brain

After the monkey learned the visually initiated, reaction-time hand movement, a localized area of the cerebral cortex was cooled or the cerebellar hemisphere was ablated to study the functional significance of the cortical area and the cerebellar hemisphere (neocerebellum) in the movement. According to many previous studies and our own investigations, we have suggested three compensatory mechanisms which follow localized lesions in the brain [21]. (1) Substitution: compensation occurring immediately through substitutional neuronal circuits. (2) Relearning: compensation by relearning through normally unused circuits. (3) Rebuilding: compensation by rebuilt neuronal circuits (sprouting and regeneration). Experimental findings suggesting the substitution and the relearning after cerebellar hemispherectomy will be briefly exemplified below [as for the rebuilding, see ref. 23].

(1) Substitution. In a monkey well trained with the visually initiated hand movement, cerebellar hemispherectomy ipsilateral to the hand downgraded the learned movement, i.e. it made the reaction time longer and more variable than before the operation. In figure 6, field potentials (S-D) recorded from the forelimb motor (FM) and somatosensory (FS) cortices before and after the operation are averaged 100 times by the stimulus onset (VS) and movement onset (LE) pulses, respectively. As seen in traces in VS averages, the operation decreased

the s-N, d-P potential in the motor cortex considerably and made reaction times longer and more variable. The LE average demonstrates that the s-N, d-P potential in the somatosensory cortex was enlarged and preceded the movement much more than before the operation. The premovement area above the baseline in the somatosensory potential is plotted on ordinate, against days after the operation on abscissa in B for three monkeys with cerebellar hemispherectomy. All the 3 cases (three different symbols) show remarkable enhancement at several days after the operation which declines within 30–40 days. This suggests that the somatosensory cortex compensates temporarily for the motor function of the motor cortex that cannot receive the motor command through the neocerebellum-thalamus [24].

Somatosensory cortex cooling at 5 days after the operation, in fact, stopped the reaction-time hand movement completely and the monkey just held the lever without responding to the light stimulus [24]. The forelimb muscles of the monkey under such conditions did not seem to be paralytic. This is different from the simultaneous cooling of both motor and somatosensory cortices which results in a complete flaccid paralysis [18]. The data appear to imply that, when disconnected from the neocerebellar input, the motor cortex cannot send the motor output to the lower center, and that the somatosensory cortex compensates immediately after the operation for the indirectly dysfunctioned ('decerebellated') motor cortex. Such a compensatory motor function of the somatosensory cortex appears to be replaced by some other compensatory function gradually developing within 30 days or so, its mechanism being not yet known. Compensatory motor function of the somatosensory cortex for the disabled motor cortex was demonstrated also by temporal local cooling of the motor cortex, directly dysfunctioned motor cortex [18].

(2) Relearning. When cerebellar hemispherectomy included both lateral and interpositus nuclei, prolonged reaction times persisted for many months, although some of other cerebellar symptoms improved to a certain extent. However, in the cases in which the operation involved the lateral nucleus but saved the interpositus, prolonged reaction times returned to the preoperative level in about 3 weeks (fig. 7) [20]. The recovery of reaction times was closely correlated with the reappearance and increase in size of the s-N, d-P potential in the forelimb motor cortex, which was entirely eliminated immediately after the cerebellar hemispherectomy. The time courses of recoveries in the po-

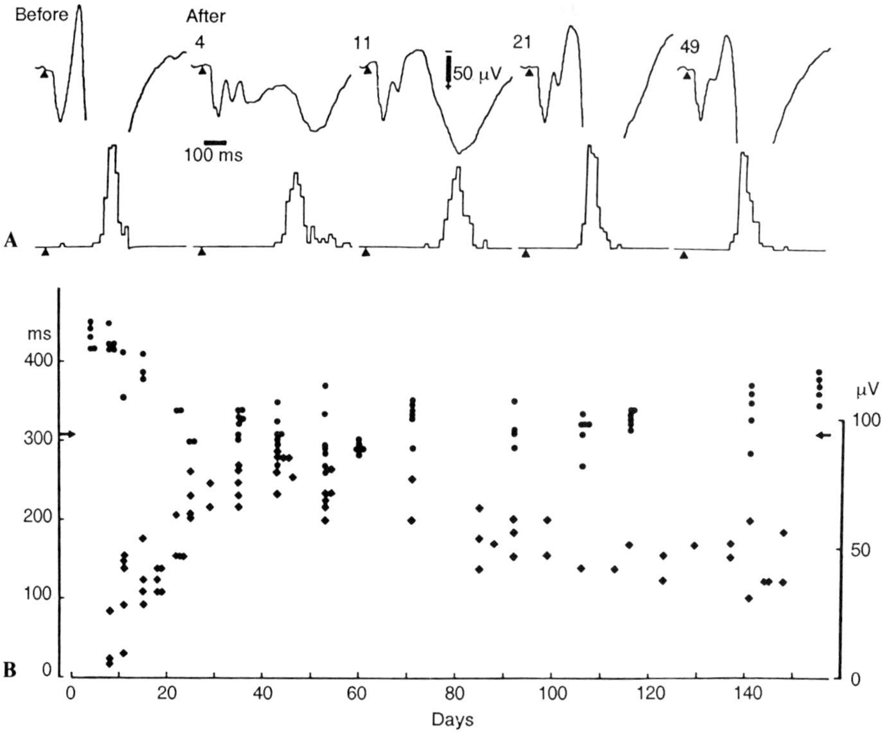

Fig. 7. **A** Visually initiated premovement potentials (S-D) in the forelimb motor cortex (upper row) and histograms of rection times (lower row) as influenced by cerebellar hemispherectomy when the interpositus nucleus was spared. Numbers indicate days after the operation. 50 μV for potentials and 100 ms for all traces. One hundred samples for every potential and histogram. **B** Reaction times (ordinate in ms to the left) (●) and the peak heights of the late s-N, d-P potentials (ordinate in μV to the right) (◆) plotted against days after cerebellar hemispherectomy (abscissa). Mean preoperative reaction time is indicated by horizontal arrows. Modified from Sasaki et al. [20].

tential and in the reaction time appear, respectively, to be similar to those of appearance of the potential and of shortening of reaction times in the process of skill learning in a normal monkey [25].

Previous microelectrophysiological studies on the cerebro-cerebellar interconnection in monkeys demonstrated that the projection area in the forelimb motor cortex from the lateral cerebellar nucleus is overlapped considerably by that from the interpositus nucleus [3]. This finding together with the results mentioned just above suggests the most reasonable explanation as follows: In a normal situation, the cerebro-cerebellar interaction for initiating the reaction-time movement includes the lateral nucleus, and the interpositus nucleus is mainly involved in some other motor control system, but when the lateral nucleus is removed or inactivated, the interpositus nucleus is utilized to replace the lateral nucleus [20]. The neuronal circuits including the interpositus nucleus will require some time for the skill learning as do those mediated by the lateral nucleus. This appears to be an example of relearning with normally unused for that purpose but existing neuronal circuits after a localized brain lesion [21].

Thalamic Action on Motor Learning and Compensation

It is interesting to note in figure 5 that the latencies of premovement potentials in various cortical areas reveal largely equal values of about 40 ms (35–47 ms) in different loci. The same order of latencies among striate (primary visual), association (prefrontal and prestriate), premotor and motor cortices suggests that impulses evoked by the visual stimulus arrive at these cortical areas almost simultaneously and in parallel when motor learning has been accomplished (fig. 5, stage IV). Also, latencies of the potentials in the respective cortical areas changed little during learning. These findings appear to imply that visually evoked impulses arrive at the primary visual cortex at the beginning of learning, simultaneously or several days later at the association and premotor cortices, then a few weeks later at the motor cortex, and thus lets the motor cortex execute the reaction time movement. At the late stage of motor learning, the cerebro-cerebellar neuronal circuits are recruited to activate the motor cortex more efficiently in order to perform the movement in fast and accurate timing skillfully.

The sequential participation of these different cortical areas with much the same latencies suggests that visually evoked impulses are conveyed in a stepwise manner to an increasing number of the different areas involved in a motor programme by a kind of 'switching' mechanism, i.e. volleys evoked by the visual stimulus are first conveyed only to the primary visual cortex, and then delivered in succession to the association and premotor cortices and later to the motor cortex. Along stages I–III of the learning process, the switching mechanism is supposed to work somewhere in the subcortical structures. The early components of premovement potentials recorded at latencies of about 40 ms in these cortices were invariably s-P, d-N ones. According to depth profiles in the cortex, they must be either due to deep T-C or C-C responses, or a mixture of both [6, 15] (fig. 1–3). Much the same latencies in the different cortices indicate that the early components are constituted mainly by deep T-C responses due to parallel projections rather than by C-C ones in serial pathways. Therefore, the switching mechanism should occur in the thalamus and/or its closely related structures [26]. Thalamic nuclei are candidates for this mechanism, since various paths of information flow, including those from the cerebral cortices, converge onto thalamic nuclei, especially association and intralaminar nuclei, which in turn project divergently onto various cortical areas directly as well as indirectly [27–30].

In processes of the substitution and relearning compensation, the same kind of switching mechanism may also occur in subcortical structures, possibly in the thalamic nuclei. For instance, when the cerebrocerebellar interaction cannot activate the motor cortex through the motor thalamic nuclei by cerebellar hemispherectomy, the motor command from the association and premotor cortices may be conveyed through other thalamic nuclei than the motor ones to the somatosensory cortex by the switching mechanisms which is immediately set on. Consequently, this cortex can send the command to the lower motor centers to execute the intended movement, although the movement is slow, weak and irregular when compared with it in the normal state (fig. 6) [18, 24]. In such a case, the cortico-thalamo-cortical interaction must have an essential role in the switching mechanism and, accordingly in compensation mechanisms.

Acknowledgements

The authors thank Prof. N. Mizuno for his help and advice on histological checking.

References

1 Sasaki K, Staunton HP, Dieckmann G: Characteristic features of augmenting and recruiting responses in the cerebral cortex. Exp Neurol 1970;26:369–392.
2 Sasaki K, Prelevic S: Excitatory and inhibitory influences of thalamic stimulation on pyramidal tract neurons. Exp Neurol 1972;36:319–335.

3 Sasaki K, Kawaguchi S, Oka H, Sakai M, Mizuno N: Electrophysiological studies on the cerebello-cerebral projections in monkeys. Exp Brain Res 1976;24:495–507.
4 Li C-L, Cullen C, Jasper HH: Laminar microelectrode analysis of cortical unspecific recruiting responses and spontaneous rhythms. J Neurophysiol 1956;19:131–143.
5 Spencer WA, Brookhart JM: Electrical patterns of augmenting and recruiting waves in depths of sensorimotor cortex of cat. J Neurophysiol 1961;24:26–49.
6 Sasaki K, Gemba H, Hashimoto S: Premovement slow cortical potentials on self-paced hand movements and thalamocortical and corticocortical responses in the monkey. Exp Neurol 1981;72:41–50.
7 Mizuno N, Mochizuki K, Akimoto C, Matsushima R, Sasaki K: Projections from the parietal cortex to the brain stem nuclei in the cat, with special reference to the parietal cerebro-cerebellar system. J Comp Neurol 1973;147:511–522.
8 Strick PL, Sterling P: Synaptic termination of afferents from the ventrolateral nucleus of the thalamus in the cat motor cortex. A light and electron microscope study. J Comp Neurol 1974;153:77–106.
9 Kawaguchi S, Samejima A, Yamamoto T: Post-natal development of the cerebello-cerebral projection in kittens. J Physiol (Lond) 1983;343:215–232.
10 Shinoda Y, Kakei S: Distribution of terminals of thalamocortical fibers originating from the ventrolateral nucleus of the cat thalamus. Neurosci Lett 1989;96:163–167.
11 Kakei S, Shinoda Y: Parietal projection of thalamocortical fibers from the ventroanterior-ventrolateral complex of the cat thalamus. Neurosci Lett 1990;117:280–284.
12 Sasaki K, Jinnai K, Gemba H, Hashimoto S, Mizuno N: Projection of the cerebellar dentate nucleus onto the frontal association cortex in monkeys. Exp Brain Res 1979;37:193–198.
13 Sasaki K, Oka H, Matsuda Y, Shimono T, Mizuno N: Electrophysiological studies of the projections from the parietal association area to the cerebellar cortex. Exp Brain Res 1975;23:91–102.
14 Sasaki K, Oka H, Kawaguchi S, Jinnai K, Yasuda T: Mossy fibre and climbing fibre responses produced in the cerebellar cortex by stimulation of the cerebral cortex in monkeys. Exp Brain Res 1977;29:419–428.
15 Sasaki K: Cerebro-cerebellar interconnections in cats and monkeys; in Massion J, Sasaki K (eds): Cerebro-Cerebellar Interaction. Amsterdam, Elsevier/North-Holland/Biomedical Press, 1979, pp 105–124.
16 Evarts EV, Thach WT: Motor mechanisms of the CNS: cerebrocerebellar interrelations. Annu Rev Physiol 1969;31:451–498.
17 Allen GI, Tsukahara N: Cerebrocerebellar communication systems. Physiol Rev 1974;54:957–1006.
18 Sasaki K, Gemba H: Compensatory motor function of the somatosensory cortex for the motor cortex temporarily impaired by cooling in the monkey. Exp Brain Res 1984;55:60–68.
19 Sasaki K, Gemba H: Development and change of cortical field potentials during learning processes of visually initiated hand movements in the monkey. Exp Brain Res 1982;48:429–437.
20 Sasaki K, Gemba H, Mizuno N: Cortical field potentials preceding visually initiated hand movements and cerebellar actions in the monkey. Exp Brain Res 1982;46:29–36.

21 Sasaki K, Gemba H: Plasticity of cortical function related to voluntary movement. Motor learning and compensation following brain dysfunction. Acta Neurochirurg 1987;(suppl 41):18–28.

22 Sasaki K, Gemba H: Effects of premotor cortex cooling upon visually initiated hand movements in the monkey. Brain Res 1986;374:278–286.

23 Kawaguchi S: Regeneration of the cerebellofugal projection after transection of the superior cerebellar peduncle in the cat. Acta Neurochirurg 1987;(suppl 41): 8–17.

24 Sasaki K, Gemba H: Compensatory motor function of the somatosensory cortex for dysfunction of the motor cortex following cerebellar hemispherectomy in the monkey. Exp Brain Res 1984;56:532–538.

25 Sasaki K, Gemba H: Learning fast and stable hand movement and cerebro-cerebellar interactions in the monkey. Brain Res 1983;277:41–46.

26 Sasaki K: Cerebro-cerebellar interactions and organization of a fast and stable hand movement: Cerebellar participation in voluntary movement and motor learning: in Bloedel JR, Dichgans J, Precht W (eds): Cerebellar Functions. Berlin, Springer, 1985, pp 70–85.

27 Hassler R: Hexapartition of input as a primary role of the thalamus; in Frigyesi T, Rinvik E, Yahr MD (eds): Corticothalamic Projections and Sensorimotor Activities. New York, Raven Press, 1972, pp 551–579.

28 Kieviet J, Kuypers HGJM: Organization of the thalamocortical connexions to the frontal lobe in the rhesus monkey. Exp Brain Res 1977;29:299–322.

29 Jones EG, Wise SP, Coulter JD: Differential thalamic relationships of sensory-motor and parietal cortical fields in monkeys. J Comp Neurol 1979;183:833–882.

30 Akert K, Hartmann-Von Monakow K: Relationships of precentral, premotor and prefrontal cortex to the mediodorsal and intralaminar nuclei of the monkey thalamus. Acta Neurobiol Exp 1980;40:7–25.

Kazuo Sasaki, MD, Department of Integrative Brain Science,
Faculty of Medicine, Kyoto University, 606 Kyoto (Japan)

Proceedings of the 2nd International Workshop on Microphysiological Recordings during Stereotactic Neurosurgery: Motor Thalamus, October 1–2, 1989, Nikko, Japan
Stereotact Funct Neurosurg 1993;60:121–126

What Goes on in the Motor Thalamus?

Ronald R. Tasker[a], *J.O. Dostrovsky*[b]

Division of Neurosurgery, Toronto Werstern Division, Toronto Hospital, Departments of [a] Surgery and [b] Physiology, University of Toronto, Ont., Canada

Key Words. Stereotactic surgery · Involuntary movements · Microelectrode recording · Stimulation · Thalamus

Abstract. Physiological observations made in man offer a unique opportunity to understand the motor thalamus. On the one hand, the patient can describe what he feels when a site is stimulated; on the other, one can observe any induced motor effect, both in 'normal' patients and in those with movement disorders. Finally, all this can be correlated with single unit recordings at the same site. Data has been correlated relative to the motor thalamus from over 10,000 macrostimulation sites and from 114 patients undergoing microstimulation and microrecording, in an attempt to understand something of the function of this part of the brain.

Introduction

Physiologic corroboration of the target site is an essential step in thalamotomy to control tremor and other dyskinesias, and can be accomplished either by macrostimulation or by microelectrode recording. After many years' experience with macrostimulation for this purpose, we summarize our experience at over 10,000 brain sites in all and with the thalamus in particular [1, 2]. We have developed a method of using microelectrodes capable of discriminating single neurons for both recording and microstimulation [3].

We have attempted to correlate macroelectrode with microelectrode data obtained in 114 patients to devise a protocol for recognition of different thalamic structures and of those involved in the lesions made to control dyskinesia. Any conclusions reached can only be tentative, since we have been able to complete physiological anatomic corre-

1011–6125/93/0603–0121 $ 2.75/0

lations in only 6 patients (only 2 with dyskinesia) after macrostimulation, none after using microelectrodes.

The Tactile Relay

Using microelectrodes in man readily identifies the tactile relay [4]. Intermixed masses of discriminated neurons are readily recorded which respond, phasically or tonically, to a variety of tactile responses – hair bending, light touch, stroking with cotton, pressure – with receptive fields (RFs) arranged somatotopographically in a more or less medial to lateral fashion, as in subhuman primates. The largest volumes of thalamus are reserved for lips and manual digits and hand, with RFs always contralateral, in our experience, as small as 2–3 mm in diameter, located in the ventrocaudal nucleus (VC). Microstimulation of such recording sites always produces paresthesiae, usually, but not always, in an area including the RFs, sometimes precisely in the RFs and with thresholds as low as 2 μA [5, 6]. Macrostimulation also induces contralateral and, especially in trigeminal territory, sometimes bilateral paresthesiae referred to larger bodily areas [1].

Spinothalamic Tract (STT)

We found no physiological evidence for spinothalamic function in VC proper, either with macro- or with microstimulation, but not yet with microelectrode recordings we have identified, in the region of VCpc, contralateral (and with macrostimulation occasionally bilateral) responses described as warm, cold, burning, or painful, not paresthetic. The somatotopy of these responses is different to that of VC proper, and in 3 patients lesions here produced dissociated sensory loss [7]. We believe our observations support Hassler's contention that this is a relay for STT [8].

Kinesthetic Relay

Immediately rostral and dorsal to neurons with tactile responses, we have found, as have others, neurons responding to passive contralateral limb movements or muscle and tendon squeezing, arranged somatotopographically medially to laterally, but less clearly so than tactile cells [4]. We believe these cells constitute the kinesthetic portion of the lemniscal relay and the spindle pathway, but, despite being able to discrimate individual neurons, are unable to distinguish the two pathways. It is our impression, like that of others, without having anatomical proof, that these so-called kinesthetic cells are located in Vim, not the VC [9–15]. In patients with tremor they constitute evoked tremor cells, and comparable dystonia cells have been recognized [9–16].

Microstimulation of these cells virtually always elicits contralateral paresthesiae in a body part related to the RF, indistinguishable from those elicited from tactile cells. However, macrostimulation in this same area occasionally produces a contralateral sensation suggestive of some motor effect, but, in the absence of such, often described as pulling, tightening, pulsing, pressure, etc., or even as a desire to move or a feeling of weakness [1, 2, 5, 6].

The Rostral Vestibular Pathway

Apparently intermingled with kinesthetic cells, we have found evidence with macrostimulation, but not yet with microstimulation, for the rostral vestibulothalamic pathway described in subhuman primates, the stimulation of which induces a feeling of faintness, nausea or vertigo [17].

The Dentatothalamic Pathway

Rostral to kinesthetic cells, we, like others, have found cells that fire in advance of a given contralateral voluntary movement, some with RFs [5, 6, 9, 14, 18, 19]. We have assumed that they represent the dentatothalamic relay destined for motor cortex, and, in patients with Parkinson's disease, they constitute the autonomous tremor cells. Both micro- and macrostimulation here often induces a muscular contraction in related body parts, very discrete or more generalized, depending on current used, at the onset of a stimulus train, different from the tetanization seen in, say, corticospinal tract or oculomotor nerve [1, 2]. We are uncertain whether these responses occur in the Vim or posterior-ventral oral nucleus (Vop).

Auditory Pathway

In the medial geniculate nucleus (MG), neurons can be found that fire in response to an auditory stimulus in the contralateral ear. Both macro- and microstimulation in MG and lateral lemniscus elicit contra- or bilateral auditory effects, often described as buzzing [1].

Other Structures

Although a variety of other structures can be recognized with macrostimulation [1], we have, as yet, not developed the means of identifying other pathways with microelectrodes.

The Target for Thalamotomy for Movement Disorder

Though other targets have been used (globus pallidus, capsule, subthalamus, dentate nucleus) thalamotomy is perhaps the commonest procedure done to control parkinsonian tremor. And although it has been suggested that lesions to control other dyskinesias should be larger or extend more rostrally than the thalamotomy lesion for tremor, still the lesion remains very similar in all these conditions.

Various criteria have been suggested for the selection of the optimal target for thalamotomy – destruction of kinesthetic cells, in keeping with the notion that tremor or other dyskinesia is the result of a disordered sensory feedback loop; of dentatothalamic cells, especially those with RFs, in keeping with the notion of that tremor is the result of a central pacemaker; sites where the most striking tremor or other dyskinesia arrest (or driving) occurs with stimulation at the lowest threshold [1, 2, 5, 6, 9–16, 20]. Moreover, it has been suggested that lesions should be made in Vim, Vop, anterior ventral oral nucleus or combinations thereof. Without the ability to carry out sophisticated neuro-anatomical studies at autopsy in patients who have been carefully explored with microelectrodes, the true target structures cannot be defined with certainty. It is even quite unclear in which nuclei the kinesthetic and dentatothalamic pathways lie.

Questions requiring answers are whether kinesthetic, dentatothalamic, and/or other structures are important; whether the entire kinesthetic or dentatothalamic array for the whole hemibody must be eliminated to stop, say, hand tremor; whether dyskinesia in both distal (digital) and proximal (shoulder) sites can be controlled; whether the extent of control possible in different dyskinesias is the same; what the relationship of complications, such as dysarthria, manual ataxia, and gait disturbance is to lesions in these pathways; whether the target is really different for different types of movement disorders, and, if so, why.

Resolution of these problems will only evolve from the pooled studies of all centres using microelectrode recordings to guide their surgery.

References

1 Tasker RR, Organ LW, Hawrylyshyn PA: The Thalamus and Midbrain of Man. A Physiological Atlas Using Electrical Stimulation. Springfield, Thomas, 1982.

2 Tasker RR, Organ LW, Hawrylyshyn P: Investigation of the surgical target for alleviation of involuntary movement disorders. Appl Neurophysiol 1982;45:261–274.

3 Lenz FA, Dostrovsky JO, Kwan HC, Tasker RR, Yamashiro K, Murphy JT: Methods for microstimulation and recording of single neurons and evoked potentials in the human central nervous system. J Neurosurg 1988;68:630–634.

4 Lenz FA, Dostrovsky JO, Tasker RR, Yamashiro K, Kwan HC, Murphy JT: Single-unit analyses of the human ventral thalamic nuclear group; somatosensory responses. J Neurophysiol 1988;59:299–316.

5 Tasker RR, Lenz FA, Dostrovsky JO, Yamashiro K, Chodakiewitz J, Albe-Fessard DG: The physiological basis of VIM thalamotomy for involuntary movement disorders; in Struppler A, Weindl A (eds): Clinical Aspects of Sensory Motor Integration. Berlin, Springer, 1987, pp 265–276.

6 Tasker RR, Yamashiro K, Lenz F, Dostrovsky JO: Thalamotomy for Parkinson's disease: Microelectrode technique; in Lunsford LD (ed): Modern Stereotactic Neurosurgery. Boston, Martinus Nijhoff, 1988, pp 297–314.

7 Tasker RR: Somatotopographic representation in the human thalamus, midbrain and spinal cord. The anatomical basis for surgical relief of pain; in Morley TP (ed): Current Controversies in Neurosurgery. Philadelphia, Saunders, 1976, pp 485–495.

8 Hassler R: Dichotomy of facial pain conduction in the diencephalon; in Hassler R, Walker AE (eds): Trigeminal Neuralgia. Pathogenesis and Pathophysiology. Stuttgart, Thieme, 1970, pp 123–138.

9 Albe-Fessard D: Electrophysiological methods for the identification of thalamic nuclei. Z Neurol 1973;205:15–28.

10 Bertrand C, Martinez SN, Hardy J, Molina-Negro P, Velasco F: Stereotactic surgery for parkinsonism. Microelectrode recording, stimulation, and oriented sections with a leucotome. Prog Neurol Surg 1973;5:79–112.

11 Crowell RM, Perret E, Siegfried J, Villoz JP: 'Movement units' and 'tremor phasic units' in the human thalamus. Brain Res 1968;11:481–488.
12 Fukamachi A, Ohye C, Narabayashi H: Delineation of the thalamic nuclei with a microelectrode in stereotaxic surgery for parkinsonism and cerebral palsy. J Neurosurg 1973;39:214–225.
13 Guiot G, Hardy J, Albe-Fessard D: Délimitation précise des structures sous-corticales et identification des noyaux thalamiques chez l'homme par l'électrophysiologie stéréotaxique. Neurochirurgia 1962;5:1–18.
14 Jasper H, Bertrand G: Thalamic units involved in somatic sensation and voluntary and involuntary movements in man; in Purpura D, Yahr M (eds): The Thalamus. New York, Columbia, 1986, pp 365–390.
15 Ohye C, Fukamachi A, Narabayashi H: Spontaneous and evoked activity of sensory neurons and their organization in the human thalamus. Z Neurol 1972;203:219–234.
16 Lenz FA, Tasker RR, Kwan HC, Schnider S, Kwong R, Murayama Y, Dostrovsky JO, Murphy JT: Single unit analysis of the human ventral thalamic nuclear group; correlation of thalamic 'tremor cells' with the 3–6 Hz component of parkinsonian tremor. J Neurosci 1988;8:754–764.
17 Hawrylyshyn PA, Rubin AM, Tasker RR, Organ LW, Fredrickson JM: Vestibulothalamic projections in man. A sixth primary sensory pathway. J Neurosphysiol 1978;41:394–401.
18 Lenz FA, Kwan HC, Dostrovsky JO, Tasker RR, Murphy JT, Lenz YE: Single unit analysis of the human ventral thalamic nuclear group. Activity correlated with movement. Brain 1990;113:1795–1821.
19 Raeva SN: Unit activity of some deep nuclear structures of the human brain during voluntary movements; in Somjen GG (ed): Neurophysiology Studied in Man. Amsterdam, Excerpta Medica, 1972, pp 64–78.
20 Lenz FA, Tasker RR, Kwan HC, Schnider S, Kwong R, Dostrovsky JO, Murphy JT: Selection of the optimal lesion site for the relief of Parkinsonian tremor on the basis of spectral analysis of neuronal firing patterns. Appl Neurophysiol 1987;50:338–343.

Ronald R. Tasker, MD, Division of Neurosurgery, Department of Surgery,
Toronto Western Hospital, University of Toronto,
399 Bathurst Street – McL 2-431, Toronto, Ontario M5T 2S8 (Canada)

Proceedings of the 2nd International Workshop on Microphysiological Recordings during Stereotactic Neurosurgery: Motor Thalamus, October 1–2, 1989, Nikko, Japan
Stereotact Funct Neurosurg 1993;60:127–134

Three-Dimensional Electrophysiological Atlas Created by Computer Mapping of Clinical Responses Elicited on Stimulation of Human Subcortical Structures

Masafumi Yoshida

Department of Neurosurgery, Kurume University School of Medicine, Kurume, Japan

Key Words. Computer · Data processing · Functional brain atlas · Neurophysiology · Parkinsonism · Stereotactic surgery · Thalamus

Abstract. A computer-generated three-dimensional functional atlas, based on clinical responses elicited upon electrical stimulation of subcortical structures of awake patients during stereotactic functional neurosurgery is presented, which shows a characteristic distribution pattern of motor, sensory and autonomic or emotional responses, respectively. The computer system used in this study is capable of accumulation and processing of data with three-dimensional coordinates, which can be converted to an anterior commissure-posterior commissure coordinate (AC-PC) system, and displays the processed data three-dimensionally together with a three-dimensional atlas created by interpolation of the Schaltenbrand-Bailey's atlas for standard anatomical landmarks.

Introduction

Among the many unique features of clinical stereotactic functional neurosurgery is the capability to obtain voluminous amounts of neurophysiological data from human subjects in the awake state. Although recent functional stereotactic neurosurgery has shifted from ablative to stimulation procedures, these intraoperative data remain as one of the

1011–6125/93/0603–0127 $ 2.75/0

most important guides for precise and optimal target localization. Since most of such data are correlated to a point which can be precisely located in a three-dimensional coordinate system, when these data are fed into computer together with corresponding three-dimensional coordinates, a huge data library harbored in a three-dimensional matrix can be created. Such data can be subject to an efficient three-dimensional analysis to be used as an intraoperative guide and for comprehensive understanding of the neurophysiology of human subcortical structures [1, 2].

In this study, sensory, motor and emotional or autonomic responses elicited on electrical stimulation of human subcortical structures are fed into a computer, and a functional atlas is created by computer mapping of these data on a three-dimensional anatomical atlas [3], which is created by interpolation from the Schaltenbrand-Bailey atlas [4].

Methods and Clinical Materials

The clinical materials consists of 14 parkinsonian, 2 tremor patients, and 2 patients with thalamic or pseudothalamic pain. The target area is determined by the nature of the disease. For parkinsonians and tremor patients, Vim is selected and for deafferentation pain syndrome, the posterior limb of the internal capsule and/or VPL is selected. For each procedure, one to three trajectories were explored for this stimulation study. Along each trajectory, in the vicinity of the target point, stimulation studies were performed at several 3-mm steps.

The stimulation electrode used in this study is a bipolar, coaxial, either stainless steel or tungsten semi-microelectrode with tip diameter of approximately 50 μm. Two mA constant current with a frequency range from 5 to 90 Hz and stimulation duration of 0.2–0.5 ms was used for electrical stimulation.

For the three-dimensional coordinate system, the one based on the anterior (AC) and posterior commissures (PC) is used. The three-dimensional coordinates of each of the stimulation points were calculated by computer using digitized information of sets of intraoperative antero-posterior and lateral X-ray films, including one visualizing the third ventricle. In this process, parallax and magnification attributable to X-ray beams, tilt and rotation of the patients' heads were taken into account.

For computer input, clinical responses elicited upon electrical stimulation of each human subcortical structure is coded by both modality and somatic representation of response. These data were grouped by response modality into three categories, i.e. sensory, motor and emotional or autonomic, and analyzed by each category.

For the anatomical atlas upon which functional data are to be displayed, a three-dimensional 0.5-mm interval atlas [3] was created by interpolation from the Schaltenbrand-Bailey atlas [4]. With this atlas any point can be displayed on an atlas which is

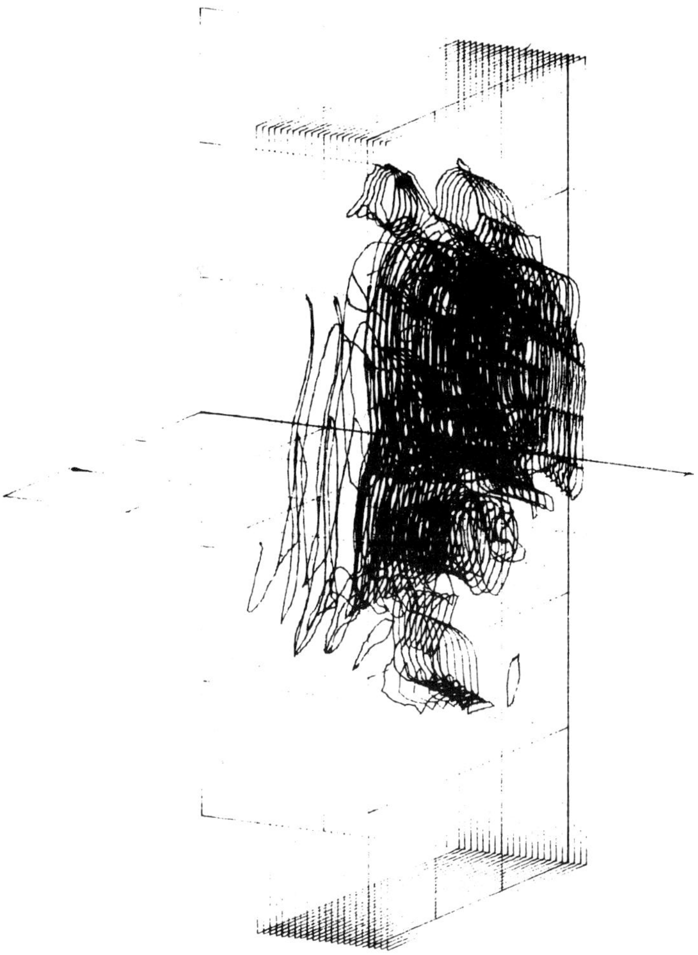

Fig. 1. Three-dimensional display of serial frontal section of 0.5 mm step atlas. Display range = Fa 1.5–Fp 9.0.

within 0.25 mm distance from that point, and the three-dimensional orientation of various structures can be more easily understood (fig. 1).

For mapping of functional data in this presentation, a set of 2 successive frontal atlas is serially displayed at intervals of 17 mm, so that, in effect, it can be seen as if 1 mm thick sliced brain is three-dimensionally displayed at appropriate interval (fig. 2–4).

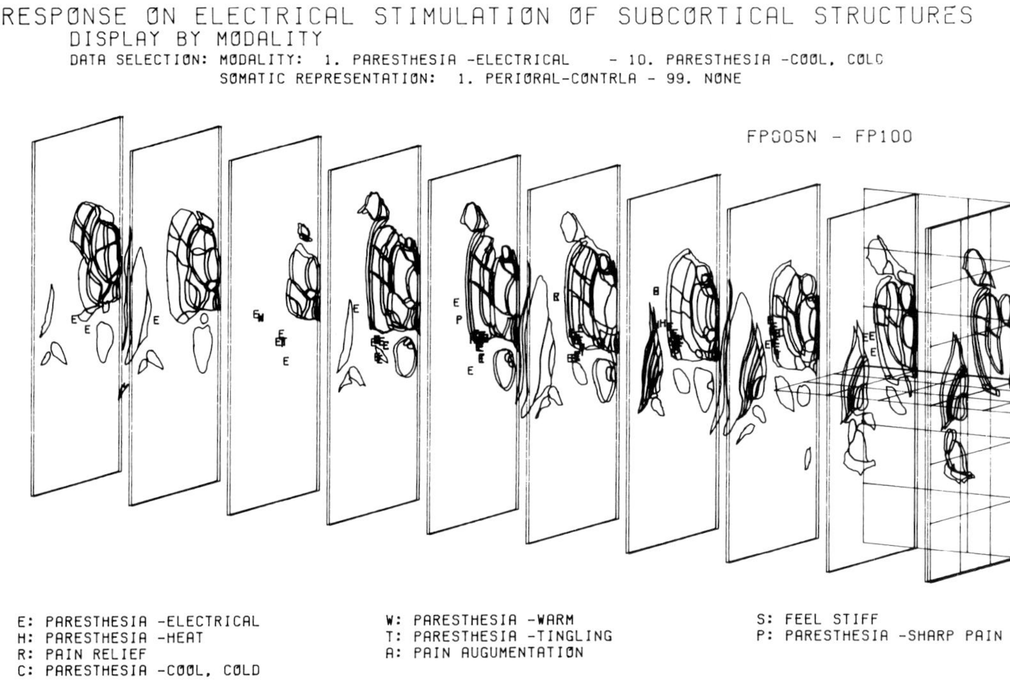

Fig. 2. Sensory responses. Response modality is coded and plotted at stimulation sites. Display range = Fp 0.5–Fp 10.0.

Results

Since subcortical targets were approached via frontal burr holes in each case, the anatomical distribution of stimulation points is confined to the location of our usual trajectory, which is directed ventro-medio-posteriorly from the frontal burr hole and most densely concentrated in the Vop and Vim areas (fig. 2–4).

Sensory responses (fig. 2): The majority of sensory responses were paresthesia of electrical sensation. The stimulation points for sensory response are widely distributed within the distribution of our trajectories. When somatic representation of sensory responses are examined (not shown), the majority represented face, hand or the upper extremity region, and only in a few stimulations was the lower limb represented. An apparent somatotopic distribution does not seem to exist.

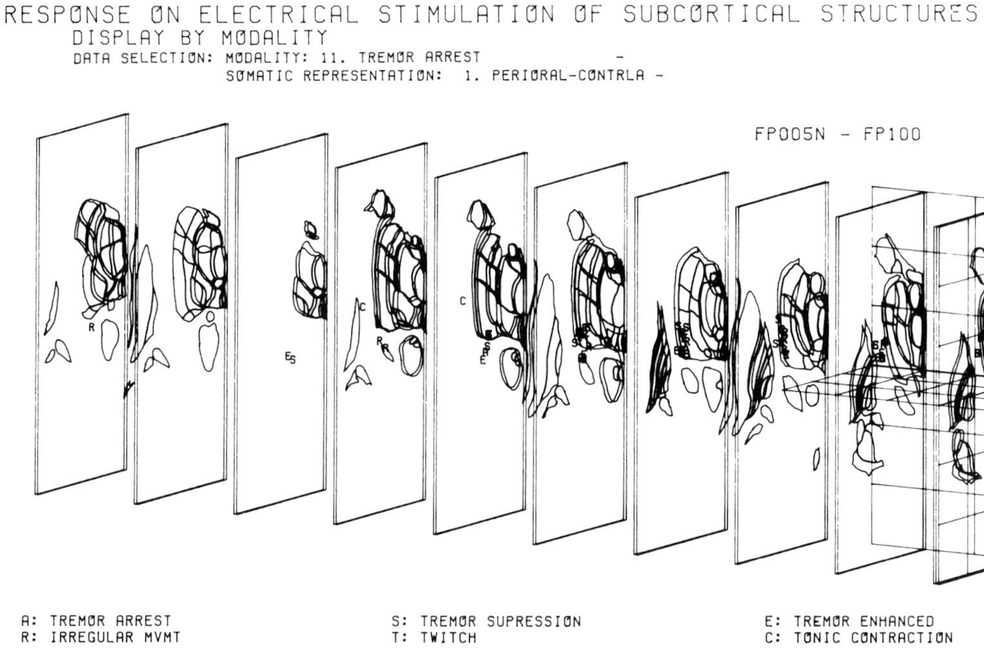

Fig. 3. Motor responses. Response modality is coded and plotted at stimulation sites. Display range = Fp 0.5–Fp 10.0.

Motor response (fig. 3): The functional atlas based on motor responses showed marked contrast to that based on sensory responses in that the points from which motor responses, were elicited were confined to the Vim and Vop areas, and also in the adjacent internal capsule. Except perhaps for irregular movement, no pure motor response was noted, and the majority were related to tremulous movement. When somatic representation is examined (not shown), they were exclusively noted in the upper limb especially the hand region. To interpret this result, one must consider that motor responses were primarily evaluated by the effect of stimulation on tremulous movement, usually noted in the upper extremity. When the motor response is examined in more detail, stimulation points for tremor arrest or suppression and those for tremor enhancement were rather widely distributed,

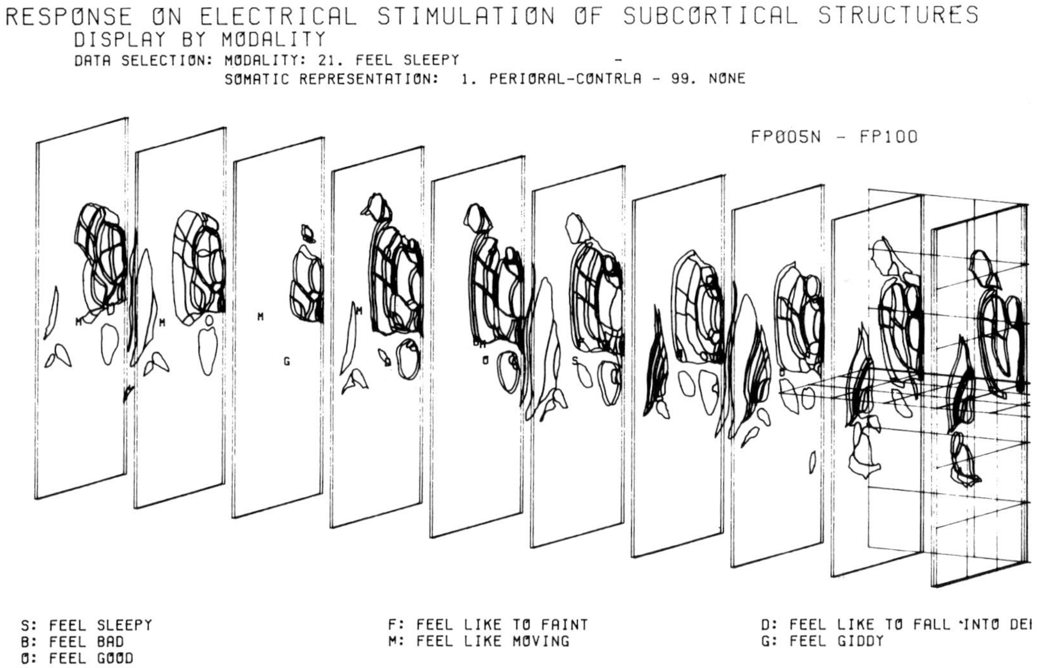

Fig. 4. Autonomic and emotional responses. Response modality is coded and plotted at stimulation sites. Display range = Fp 0.5–Fp 10.0.

whereas irregular movement of the hand was noted in a rather confined area in the lateral portion of Vim and Vop, which seemed to be closely related to the adjacent reticular nucleus.

Emotional, autonomic and other responses (fig. 4): Responses in this category, some of which were difficult to classify, were elicited upon stimulation of rather wide areas, but they are primarily noted in the subthalamic field or in the upper midbrain.

Discussion

The advantage of this sort of study is that the data obtained are from human subjects in the awake state. Since these data are voluminous and precisely correlated to three-dimensional localizable points in the human brain, computer-assisted data processing is best suited for comprehensive analysis [1, 2]. On the other hand, there are disadvantages, primarily attributed to the limits of the clinical setting in the operating room. The sites from which data are obtained are limited, i.e. the stimulation area in this study is confined to the vicinity of the ventral and lateral tiers of the thalamus, and more detailed neurophysiological studies are not possible. However, points from which sensory, motor and autonomic or emotional responses are elicited show a rather characteristic distribution pattern. In particular the 'functional motor thalamus' was delineated by motor responses, mostly related to tremulous movement, and was well localized in the ventrolateral region of the thalamus. Furthermore, irregular movement was noted in a rather confined area in the lateral aspect of the Vim and Vop and the adjacent internal capsule.

Somatic representation of currently explored stimulation points was noted to be primarily hand, upper limb, face and trunk in sensory response and exclusively hand in motor response. No characteristic somatotopic pattern was noted.

The computer system used in this study is capable of accumulation and processing of all kinds of data which come with three-dimensional coordinates which can be converted to an anterior commissure-posterior commissure coordinate (AC-PC) system. The results are displayed in three-dimensions together with a three-dimensional atlas created by interpolation of the Schaltenbrand-Bailey atlas for standard anatomical landmarks.

Various schemes of such data in the form of three-dimensional voxel data are now widely available. They include voxel data from CT scans, magnetic resonance (MR) imaging and positron emission tomography (PET). These data obtained noninvasively, are individualized to each patient, and cover all cranial and intracranial structures.

In present CT scanners, voxel size can be small enough to localize fine structures, including AC and PC. Since three-dimensional coordinates of structures visualized by CT images are precise, by direct reading of three-dimensional coordinates of AC and PC, conversion of CT data to an AC-PC coordinate system is possible [5].

MR imaging with superior resolution can visualize more detail of anatomy, but its spatial accuracy is somewhat less than of CT scan. In PET, three-dimensional voxel data are of low resolution and accurate localization of cerebral reference points is difficult. However, since voxel data of MR imaging and PET are obtained with essentially the same principle as those of CT scans, with use of localizer (or mechanical interface) which can, preferably noninvasively, be securely fixed to the patient's head and be visualized precisely in all CT, MR and PET images, three-dimensional coordinates of cerebral reference points can be localized on voxel data of CT, MR imaging and PET by the position of the localizer interface. Thus, three-dimensional voxel data of MRI and PET can be precisely reformatted to be aligned to the AC-PC coordinate system. Therefore, similar to the functional atlas described above, an anatomical or functional (or neurochemical) atlas, based on various filtered or unfiltered image data, can be displayed together with a three-dimensional anatomical atlas [5]. In both instances, simultaneous display of neurophysiological data obtained during stereotactic functional surgery is possible.

This approach means integration of (1) intraoperatively obtained neurophysiological data from a group of patients who underwent stereotactic functional neurosurgery; (2) noninvasively obtained morphological (CT scan and MR imaging) and biochemical (PET) data both from a control group and from patients with a wide range of pathology, and (3) microscopic anatomy, as defined by cytoarchitecture.

We believe that further accumulation of this sort of information will be valuable in understanding the functional organization of deep subcortical structures and will be useful for optimal target localization during various stereotactic functional neurosurgical procedures.

References

1 Tasker RR, Organ LW, Hawrylyshyn P: The Thalamus and Midbrain of Man. A Physiological Atlas Using Electrical Stimulation. Springfield, Thomas, 1982.
2 Yoshida, M: Mapping of semi-microelectrode stimulation response in and around the thalamus. Stereotact Funct Neurosurg 1989;52:171–175.
3 Yoshida M: Creation of a three-dimensional atlas by interpolation from Schaltenbrand-Bailey's atlas. Appl Neurophysiol 1987;50:45–48.
4 Schaltenbrand G, Bailey P (eds): Introduction to Stereotaxis with an Atlas of Human Brain. Stuttgart, Thieme, 1959.
5 Kall BA, Kelly PJ, Goerss S, Frieder G: Methodology and clinical experience with computed tomography and a computer-resident stereotactic atlas. Neurosurgery 1985;17:400–407.

Masafumi Yoshida, MD, Department of Neurosurgery,
Kurume University School of Medicine, 67 Asahi-machi, Kurume, 830 (Japan)

Proceedings of the 2nd International Workshop on Microphysiological Recordings during Stereotactic Neurosurgery: Motor Thalamus, October 1–2, 1989, Nikko, Japan
Stereotact Funct Neurosurg 1993;60:135

Animal Models of Tremor: Thalamo-Cortical and Olivo-Cerebellar Generators

Y. Lamarre
Université de Montréal, Canada

From several experimental approaches (brain lesions, electrophysiological recordings and the use of tremorgenic drugs) three types of experimental tremor can be distinguished in the monkey. One type (8–12 Hz) appears in normal animals following harmaline injection and is characterized by synchronous activation of antagonistic muscle pairs. It is produced by the olivo-cerebellar system and is regarded as a model of physiological tremor. Another type showing the characteristics of human essential tremor (6–8 Hz) is also produced by the olivo-cerebellar system, but appears only in monkeys with lesion of the cerebellar nuclei and harmaline stimulation. The third type is a model of parkinsonian tremor (4–6 Hz) and occurs spontaneously in monkeys following lesions of the ventromedial tegmentum of the midbrain. This tremor appears to be generated at the thalamo-cortical level. The tremor mechanisms at the level of the olivo-cerebellar system could involve a gaba-ergic system controlling electrotonic coupling between olivary neurons. Similar mechanisms can be postulated at the level of the motor thalamus.

1011–6125/93/0603–0135 $ 2.75/0

Proceedings of the 2nd International Workshop on Microphysiological Recordings during Stereotactic Neurosurgery: Motor Thalamus, October 1–2, 1989, Nikko, Japan
Stereotact Funct Neurosurg 1993;60:136–145

Tremor-Mediating Thalamic Zone Studied in Humans and in Monkeys

C. Ohye, T. Shibazaki, T. Hirai, Y. Kawashima, M. Hirato, M. Matsumura

Department of Neurosurgery, Gunma University School of Medicine, Gunma, Japan

Key Words. Tremor · Thalamus · Human · Rhythmic burst · Microrecording · Monkey · Stereotactic surgery

Abstract. The thalamic zone mediating the rhythmic burst activity related to the contralateral tremor was studied by microelectrodes in clinical cases with tremor and in monkeys with experimental tremor. The rhythmic burst time-locked with the tremor was found in a restricted area of the ventrointermedius nucleus (Vim) in humans and also in VPLo nucleus in monkeys. In both cases, only the lateral and ventrocaudal part of each nucleus, which was defined as the kinesthetic zone, was involved. A possible tremor-mediating neural circuit is postulated.

Introduction

Using microelectrodes, we have been recording rhythmic discharge time-locked with the peripheral tremor within the human thalamus [1–3]. This is important for the therapeutic purpose of stereotactic thalamotomy, because a small coagulation including this thalamic point results in almost permanent arrest of the tremor of whatever kind [4, 5]. In a series of some 300 cases, we have recorded substantial numbers of rhythmic grouped discharges in the human thalamus, mostly in patients with Parkinson's disease. Interesting enough, the tremor-related rhythmic discharges were clustered in a certain restricted area of the ventrointermediate nucleus (Vim).

1011–6125/93/0603–0136 $ 2.75/0

Also, in experimental tremor in monkeys, we tried to record rhythmic discharges in the corresponding area of the thalamus [6, 7], and were able to record the same rhythmic discharges as in human cases. Together with other experimental data, a hypothesis involving a tremor-mediating circuit, including the ventrointermediate nucleus, is presented.

Recording from the Human Thalamus

Using Leksell's stereotactic apparatus, usually two microelectrodes are introduced in parallel to the sagittal plane toward the tentative target point, which is 5 mm anterior to the posterior commissure, 15–17 mm lateral to the midline and on the intercommissural line, for the anteriorly positioned electrode. This tentative target point is chosen so that at least one of the electrodes would probably penetrate the Vim nucleus. In fact, in our anterolateral to posteromedial approach, which is inclined about 20° anteriorly in lateral view, the posterior electrode has more chance to pass through the Vim nucleus for a distance of 10 mm, which is consistent with the configuration of the Vim nucleus [8]. In contrast, the anterior electrode arrives at the Vim nucleus only by the end of tracking, as illustrated in figure 1.

A pair of recording electrodes is introduced with a micromanipulator (stepwise motor drive) especially adapted to Leksell's apparatus. The electrode is a concentric bipolar needle type with an outer diameter of 0.3 mm, interpolar distance of about 0.5 mm, an electrical resistance of about 100 kΩ.

Coming into the thalamus, which is indicated by increased background activity with a high cracking noise, we look for unitary or distinguishable multiunitary spike activity. In cases with resting tremor of Parkinson's disease, a rhythmic burst activity time-locked with contralateral peripheral tremor is often found (fig. 2A). An audio monitor facilitates distinguishing the rhythmic burst from the background noise. In general, such rhythmic activity is encountered in the last 10 mm of tracking, mostly from the posterior electrode, as mentioned above. When rhythmic burst activity is heard on the audio monitor, the electrodes are introduced carefully with shorter steps to identify a stable spike activity by using a micromanipulator.

Whenever a stable spike discharge is recorded, an attempt is made

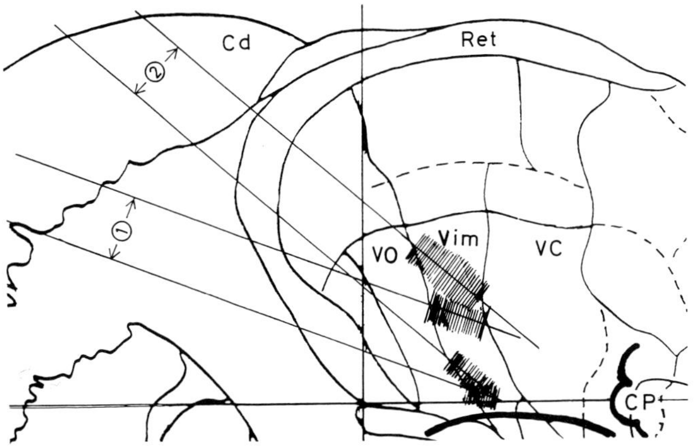

Fig. 1. Sagittal view of the lateral thalamus containing VO (ventrooral nucleus), vim (ventrointermediate nucleus) and VC (ventrocaudal nucleus), with a part of caudate (Cd) nucleus. Relative relation of Vim nucleus and the electrode tracking (oblique lines, 1 and 2) are illustrated. Hatched area along the electrode indicates penetration through the Vim zone.

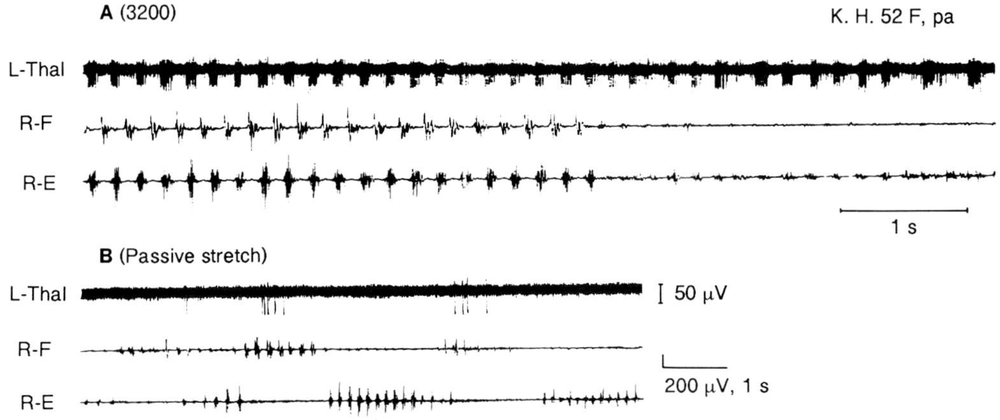

Fig. 2. Rhythmic bursting discharge recorded in a case of Parkinson's disease. **A** Thalamic discharge (uppermost trace) time-locked with peripheral tremor shown by EMG (lower two traces). Note that the rhythm in the thalamus became slightly irregular with decreased peripheral tremor rhythm. **B** The same thalamic spike responding to passive stretch of the forearm flexor muscle (F), but not to the extensor muscle (E).

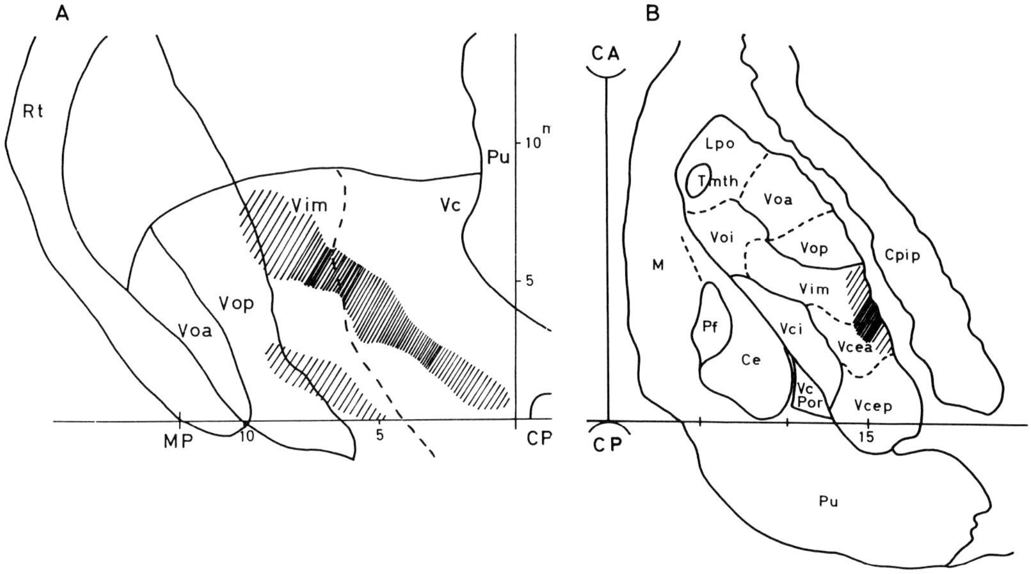

Fig. 3. Approximate extent of the ventrolateral thalamic zone where a rhythmic burst time-locked with tremor is recorded. **A** Sagittal view. **B** Horizontal view. Because of the preferential tracking by a pair of microelectrodes, all ventrolateral thalamic areas are not evenly explored.

to activate the spikes by peripheral natural stimuli, such as cutaneous touch, muscle compression, and active or passive movement of an extremity. As far as tested, it is almost always the case that the same rhythmic burst spike activity also responds to passive or active movement around a certain joint (fig. 2B). As reported previously [2, 3], in such cases, the adequate stimulus is movement related or strong compression of the involved muscle, but not light cutaneous touch. In this sense, we defined it as a kinesthetic response, the origin of which is assumed to be mostly from muscle spindles.

The distribution of the kinesthetic response, which is almost equal to the distribution of rhythmic burst activity, is limited to a certain area of the Vim and its adjacent area. As recently reconfirmed, it is the lateralmost part of the Vim nucleus, scattering dorsoventrally along the most posterior part of the ventrocaudal nucleus (fig. 3), judged from the position of the electrode tip in relation to the third ventricle on X-

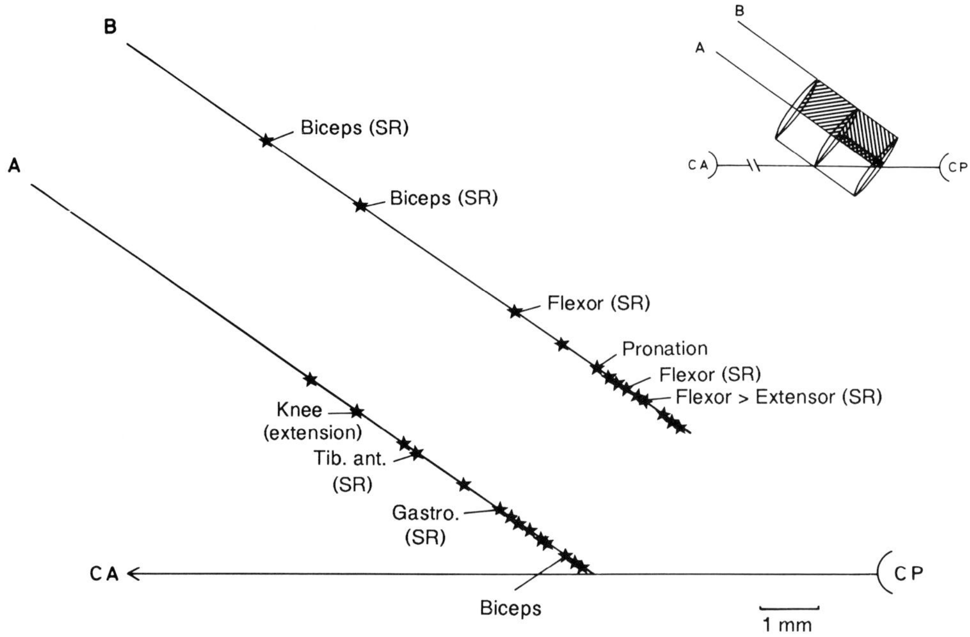

Fig. 4. An example of a thalamic recording in a case of Parkinson's disease where a cluster of rhythmic burst discharges (recording points indicated by stars) was found. Most responded also to passive stretch (SR) of body part indicated. Lateral view with the intercommissural line (horizontal line) anterior (CA), and posterior commissures (CP). Oblique lines are tracts of a pair of recording electrodes (A and B). Right upper, the coagulated areas (hatched) are illustrated in the same way, referring to the intercommissural line.

ray film. It should be mentioned that in the latter area of the Vc nucleus, the kinesthetic response never intermingles with the response of cutaneous origin, which is encountered further posterior to the kinesthetic zone in any given case.

The rhythmic burst activity is found more frequently in the ventral and lateral Vim. In a particular case with Parkinson's disease (fig. 4) recording tracking was relatively lateral because of the small third ventricular size. Along the anteroposteriorly situated parallel tracking, we found much rhythmic burst activity along about a 10-mm trajectory. Mostly, the burst activities were recorded independently by two electrodes, but at several points two different bursts appeared at the same time. They were not synchronized, in general, but some seemed to be beating simultaneously, as if they belonged to the same neuronal origin. After recording, therapeutic coagulation was made, including all these points of burst activities, and tremor of the contralateral side disappeared immediately without any side effect.

Experimental Tremor in Monkeys

Resting tremor resembling that in Parkinson's disease can be produced by a restricted coagulation of the ventromedial tegmental area involving the parvocellular red nucleus and its ventral part close to the substancia nigra [9–12]. The tremor appears usually in a week or 10 days after the coagulation on the contralateral extremities. Severity and constancy of the tremor are variable, depending on subtle differences of coagulation site and size. Our longest record of continuous resting tremor was for more than 3 years.

Once tremor is established, recordings were made along the neuroaxis, looking for rhythmic burst activity time-locked with tremor [7, 11, 13]. (Results obtained from the spinal cord level were already reported [13].) Rhythmic burst activity representing an efferent signal was found in the anterior funicule, corresponding to the pontine reticulospinal tract, ipsilateral to the peripheral tremor.

In 5 cases, recordings were also made from the thalamus contralateral to the peripheral tremor, just as in the human cases. An anterolateral to posteromedial oblique approach from the prefrontal area toward the ventroposterior lateral oral nucleus (VPLo, nonhuman primate equivalent of ventrointermedius nucleus) was used. Also, in monkey thalamus, a relatively high background activity zone was distinguished, which corresponds to the anatomically defined VPLo. In this area, rhythmic burst activity time-locked with the contralateral tremor was recorded (fig. 5). The spike discharges composed of the rhythmic discharge also responded to natural stimuli, such as passive movement or compression of the corresponding muscle belly, but not to light touch on the skin surface. In this sense, it was kinesthetic in nature. Further, electrical stimulation of the forelimb muscle involved with tremor or provoking a kinesthetic thalamic response produced excitation of the same spike discharge. The latency was variable, between 4.5 and 11 ms.

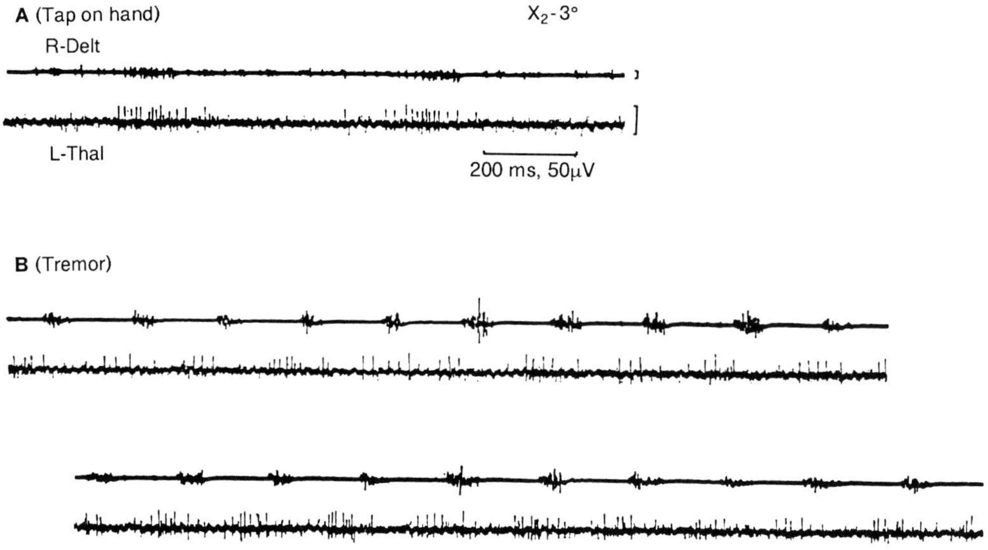

Fig. 5. **A** A kinesthetic response in the monkey thalamus (2nd trace) to a passive movement of deltoid muscle (1st trace). **B** The same spike discharge shown in **A**, now exhibiting rhythmic discharges time-locked with the spontaneous tremor.

In 2 cases, when a kinesthetic response was obtained, using an Elgyloi electrode, the recorded point was marked electrolytically by passing an electric current, and later the ferricianate deposit was stained. The marked point was found at the caudal and ventral borders of large-celled VPLo, as expected.

In order to elucidate a possible ascending pathway toward the thalamic kinesthetic zone, the effect of spinal cord dissection was tested. Bilateral dorsal column section at a high cervical level did not affect the thalamic response to electrical stimulation. In another case, it was verified that, after hemisection of the spinal cord contralateral to the thalamus, thus ipsilateral to electrical stimulation, the kinesthetic response remained (fig. 6). This suggests that a crossed spinal pathway, the spinothalamic tract, may be used as an ascending pathway for transmission of kinesthetic sensation as well as the bursting signal from trembling muscle.

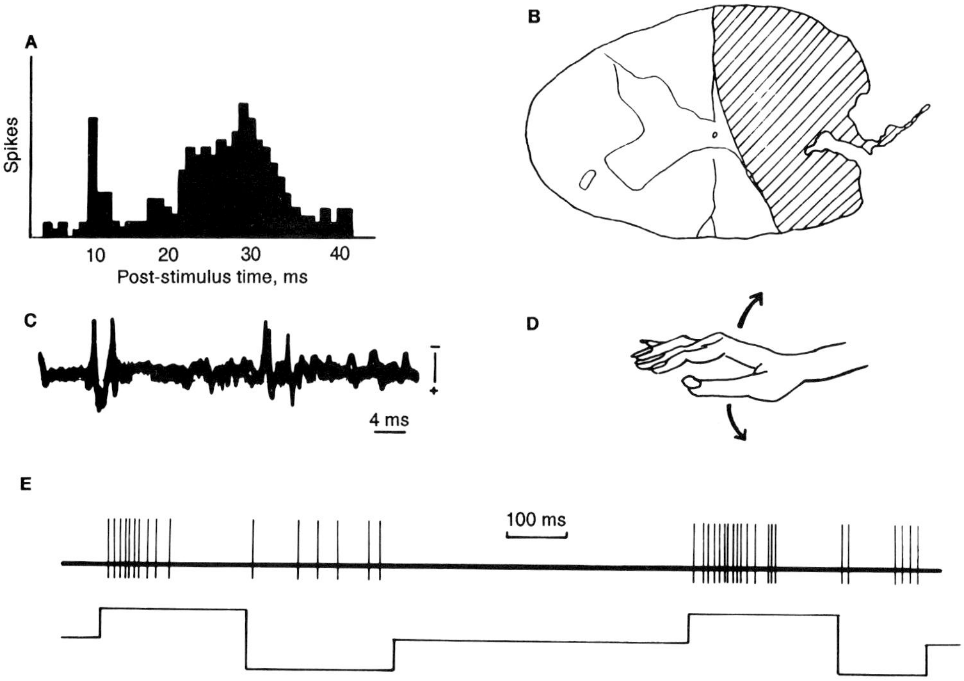

Fig. 6. **A** Poststimulus histogram showing a kinesthetic response in the monkey thalamus. **C**. An example of the response to electrical stimulation of the flexor muscle. **E** Responses to natural stimuli shown in **D**. **B** Spinal hemisection hatched area.

Discussion

Observations in human cases and experimental studies in monkeys presented here are compatible and complementary data. Rhythmic burst discharges time-locked with contralateral peripheral tremor are recorded in a restricted area of the thalamus, the lateralmost and caudal part of Vim in humans with various kinds of tremor and in monkeys with experimental tremor. There are several reasons (physiological and histological) to believe that this area is a part of the large-celled and cell sparse zone of Vim in humans [3, 14] and VPLo in monkeys [15], where kinesthetic sensation from the contralateral periphery, probably from the muscle spindle, is thought to project. Therefore, it is not surprising that signals originated from trembling muscles are found in the form of rhythmic bursting activity.

It is interesting to note that after Vim coagulation, most of the patients complain of a feeling of lightness in the operated limbs. As the responsible Vim area is the projection zone of kinesthetia, disturbance of deep sense may occur. At present, we do not know why the feeling of lightness subsides within several weeks.

The clinical implication of the physiological identification of the kinesthetic zone is unequivocal. After identifying rhythmic bursting activity or a kinesthetic response, a small coagulation including this point results in almost constant relief of the tremor of whatever cause. The only difference is the amount of coagulation volume necessary for complete arrest of tremor, dependling on the cause of tremor. Usually, Parkinson's tremor and essential tremor are abolished by a minimal lesion of about 40–60 mm^3, while coarse post-traumatic tremor and post-stroke tremor require larger lesions, sometimes exceeding 100 mm^3 [15]. In either case, the therapeutic lesion is confined within the physiologically defined Vim nucleus, which is certainly an important component of the motor thalamus [17–19].

Integrating together the present observations and knowledge about tremor, a working hypothesis has been proposed to understand the tremor-mediating neuronal circuit [20]. Once the tremor rhythm starts somewhere in the neural axis (not yet clarified), it is transferred to the peripheral muscle via the pontine reticulospinal tract (ipsilateral to the peripheral tremor). Then, the tremor signal, probably from the muscle spindle ascends the spinal cord contralateral to the tremor via the spinothalamic tract toward the thalamic Vim nucleus. Within the Vim nucleus, there is a particular structural mechanism, involving lamellar organization [15], by which the bursting discharge is synchronized and reinforced, and further transmitted to the cerebral cortex, probably to area 3a. Closing this neuronal loop, there should be a connection between 3a to the contralateral pontine reticular formation, which should be verified in the future.

References

1 Ohye C, Albe-Fessard D: Rhythmic discharges related to tremor in humans and monkeys; in Chalazonitis S: Abnormal Neuronal Discharges. New York, Raven Press, 1978, pp 37–48.
2 Ohye C, Narabayashi H: Physiological study of presumed ventralis intermedius nucleus in the human thalamus. J Neurosurg 1979;50:290–297.
3 Ohye C, Shibazaki T, Hirai T, Wada H, Hirato M, Kawashima Y: Further physio-

logical observations on the ventralis intermedius neurons in the human thalamus. J Neurophysiol 1989;61:488–500.
4 Ohye C: Selective thalamotomy for movement disorder: Microrecording, stimulation techniques and results; in Lunsford LD (ed): Textbook of Modern Stereotactic Surgery. Boston, Martinus Nijhoff, 1988, pp 315–331.
5 Nagaseki Y, Shibazaki T, Hirai T, Kawashima Y, Hirato M, Wada H, Miyazaki M, Ohye C: Long-term follow up after selective VIM-thalamotomy. J Neurosurg 1986;65:296–302.
6 Ohye C: Studies on experimental tremor (in Japanese); in Sasaki K, Hongo T (eds): Handbook of Physiology, vol 10. Tokyo, Igakushoin, 1988, pp 243–258.
7 Shibazaki T, Hirai T, Nagaseki Y, Wada H, Hirato M, Kawashima Y, Ohye C: Ascending pathways to kinesthetic neurons in the monkey thalamus. Neurosci Lett 1984;(suppl 17):S154.
8 Hassler R: In Schaltenbrand G, Wahren W (eds): Atlas for Stereotaxy of the Human Brain, ed 2. Stuttgart, Thieme, 1977.
9 Poirier LJ, Bouvier G, Bedard P, Boucher R, Larochelle L, Olivier A, Singh P: Essai sur les circuits neuronaux impliqués dans le tremblement postural et l'hyperkinésie. Rev Neurol 1969;120:15–40.
10 Larochelle L, Bedard P, Boucher R, Poirier LJ: The rubro-olivo-cerebello-rubral loop and postural tremor in the monkey. J Neurol Sci 1970;11:53–64.
11 Ohye C, Imai S, Nakajima H, Shibazaki T, Hirai T: Experimental study of spontaneous postural tremor induced by a more successful tremor-producing procedure in the monkey. Adv Neurol 1979;24:83–91.
12 Ohye C, Shibazaki T, Hirai T, Wada H, Kawashima Y, Hirato M, Matsumura M: A special role of the parvocellular red nucleus in lesion-induced spontaneous tremor in monkeys. Behav Brain Res 1988;28:241–243.
13 Ohye C, Shibazaki T, Hirai T, Nagaseki Y, Wada H, Kawashima Y, Hirato M: Possible descending pathway mediating spontaneous tremor in monkeys. Adv Neurol 1984;40:181–188.
14 Hirai T, Ohye C, Nagaseki Y, Matsumura M: Cytometric analysis of the thalamic ventralis intermedius nucleus in humans. J Neurophysiol 1989;61:478–487.
15 Jones EG: The Thalamus. New York, Plenum Press, 1985.
16 Hirai T, Miyazaki M, Nakajima H, Shibazaki T, Ohye C: The correlation between tremor characteristics and predicted volume of effective lesions in stereotaxic Vim-thalamotomy. Brain 1983;106:1001–1018.
17 Ohye C: Neurons of the thalamic ventralis intermedius nucleus. Their special reference to tremor (Japanese). Adv Neurol Sci 1985;29:222–231.
18 Ohye C: Motor disturbances by thalamic lesion. Motor thalamus. Adv Neurol Sci 1988;32:498–508.
19 Ohye C: The Thalamus; in Paxinos G (ed): The Human Nervous System. New York, Academic Press, 1990, pp 439–468.
20 Ohye C: Neurol circuits involved in parkinsonian motor disturbance studied in monkeys. Eur Neurol 1987;26(suppl 1):41–46.

C. Ohye, MD, Department of Neurosurgery, Gunma University
School of Medicine, 3-39 Showa-machi, Maebashi, Gunma (Japan)

Proceedings of the 2nd International Workshop on Microphysiological Recordings during Stereotactic Neurosurgery: Motor Thalamus, October 1–2, 1989, Nikko, Japan
Stereotact Funct Neurosurg 1993;60:146

Micro- and Semi-Microrecordings in the Ventral Thalamus of Human Patients and Monkeys with Dyskinesias

D.M. Gao[a], *L. Jeaugey*[a], *S. Lavallee*[b], *D. Hoffmann*[a], *P. Pollak*[b], *A.L. Benabid*[a]
Departments of [a] Clinical and Biological Neurosciences (INSERM U-318) and [b] Biomathematics, University of Grenoble, La Tronche, France

Chronic stimulation of the Vim nucleus has been proven to selectively suppress parkinsonian and essential tremors. This effect is frequency dependent and is more efficient at high (130 Hz) than at low (65 Hz) frequencies. The mechanism by which this effect is achieved is not understood, but could be a jamming of a feedback loop impinged on the motor pathways, as well as a specific action on an inhibitory system or group of cells. In order to further understand these events, we undertook an electrophysiological study, using microelectrode recording in the *Macacus cynomolgus* and a semi-microelectrode study in human patients during surgery for tremor. In the monkey, under ketamine anesthesia, cells responded to superficial low threshold stimuli, to deep muscular and joint inputs or to both. The somatotopy of these various types of cells was drawn according to the bicommissural reference system obtained by opaque contrast ventriculography. The corresponding areas are arranged posterior to anterior and inferior to superior in a pattern opposite to that observed in humans. Some preliminary results are obtained in MPTP-treated monkeys. In human patients, multiunits were recorded with a Ohye semi-microelectrode which allowed recording of 'neural noise' and to help locate the Vim cells. They made it possible to stimulate at each recording site and to map more closely the 'active area' where suppression of the tremor could be elicited. This area appears to be limited very closely at the level of the bicommissural line, between the second and third twelfths, of this line ahead of the posterior commissure. This should allow one to determine precisely the target of implantation of stimulating electrodes and to achieve the desired therapeutic effect with the fewest side effects.

1011–6125/93/0603–0146 $ 2.75/0

Proceedings of the 2nd International Workshop on Microphysiological Recordings during Stereotactic Neurosurgery: Motor Thalamus, October 1–2, 1989, Nikko, Japan
Stereotact Funct Neurosurg 1993;60:147–151

Thalamic Neuronal Populations Responding Selectively to Remembered Words

Yu. L. Gogolitsin, V.B. Nechaev

Institute of the Human Brain, St. Petersburg, Russia

Key Words. Neuronal activity · Lexical processing · Thalamic nuclei · Mental processes · Implanted electrodes · Neuronal detector · Memory · Neuropsychology

Abstract. In 16 Parkinson patients treated with implanted electrodes, the multi-unit impulse activity of 165 neuronal populations was recorded as a part of the diagnostic procedures during the performance of a set of verbal psychological tests. 10 neuronal populations in the thalamus revealed selective responses to visual presentation of the target words remembered prior to the test or to the presentation of both the target words and of the words closely resembling the targets graphically.

Introduction

In a previous publication, a class of neuronal reactions was described, which reflect the activity of the brain mechanisms associated with inner speech. Within the scope of the same study, another type of selective neuronal evoked reactions was also revealed in certain neuronal populations of the thalamus and striopallidal nuclei. These reactions were observed in the psychological test where the patient first had to remember two verbal stimuli (targets) and after that to discriminate them presented visually among others in a sequence.

1011–6125/93/0603–0147 $ 2.75/0

Subjects and Methods

This study was performed under the same conditions and with the same subjects as the previous one [1]. The psychological test consisted of a sequence of 144–256 trials with visual presentation to the subject of a single verbal stimulus in each trial. A computer-controlled projection tachistoscope was used to project slides on an opaque 0.8 × 0.5 m screen installed in front of the subject at a distance of 2 m. Each slide contained a sequence of five white letters on a black background, which either formed a meaningful Russian word or appeared to be a word-like meaningless sequence called quasiword. Words and quasiwords were presented in random order replacing for 100 ms a slide with a white circle in the center, which was projected for the rest of the time to provide gaze fixation.

Prior to the presentation, the subject was given two stimuli to remember (targets), usually one meaningful word and one quasiword. He was instructed to respond 'yes' to these stimuli only and 'no' to all other verbal stimuli presented in a sequence.

The set of verbal stimuli was intentionally selected in such a way that among non-targets there were words and quasiwords clearly graphically similar to the targets but clearly different (e.g. four letters of five are the same and in the same positions).

Neuronal reactions to verbal stimuli were assessed by constructing and statistically comparing the peri-stimulus-time histograms of multiunit activity for the groups of trials with targets, similar non-targets and different non-targets presented.

Results

Figure 1 shows a typical example of the selective reaction to remembered verbal stimuli. It can be clearly seen that presentation of the target stimuli only elicits in this neuronal population a statistically significant short phasic reaction in that the discharge rate increased with a latency of around 450 ms. Presentation of the non-targets, words and quasiwords, both similar and dissimilar, did not result in the appearance of such a discharge rate peak.

Another example (fig. 2) demonstrates a response component appearing with approximately the same latency after both targets (M1) and graphically similar non-targets (M2) were shown, and the absence of this component in trials with presentation of the dissimilar non-targets (M3). It should be noted that, in the two latter cases (M2 and M3), the subject always uttered 'no' after the presentation of the slide, so the difference between M2 and M3 cannot be explained in terms of the possible influence of difference in the verbal response.

Thirty-six neuronal populations (among 165 studied) revealed similar properties of the evoked neuronal reactions to discrimination of

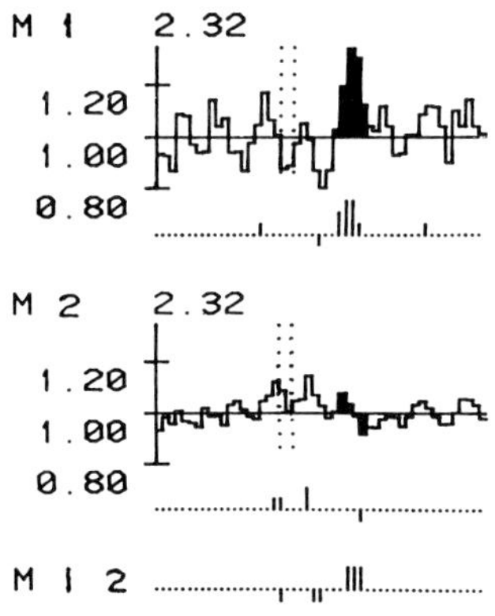

Fig. 1. Discharge rate of the neuronal population in the ZI of the right hemisphere recorded during discrimination of the remembered verbal stimuli. Each graph shows a peri-stimulus-time histogram (PSTH) with 50 ms time bins. Relative discharge rate deviation is plotted along the vertical axis. The unit level corresponds to the population background mean rate (absolute values given in spikes per bin above the graphs). The horizontal dotted line under the graph shows single time bins and is used to mark those with contents deviating significantly (t criterion) from the background mean value. Short, medium and long bar markers correspond to $p < 0.05$, $p < 0.01$ and $p < 0.001$ confidence levels. Double dotted vertical lines denote the presentation epoch for the slide containing the processed stimulus. M1 = PSTH for the trials where targets were presented; M2 = PSTH for the trials with non-targets presented; M1 2 = results of the pairwise statistical bin comparison of M1 and M2.

remembered verbal stimuli, 10 located in the thalamic nuclei, 11 in the striopallidal system with 27 of 36 in the left hemisphere.

Fifteen of 36 neuronal populations demonstrated clear phasic reactions to the target presentation only, but did not respond to the presentation of any non-targets, whereas the remaining 21 revealed statistically significant responses both to presentation of the remembered targets and graphically similar non-target verbal stimuli.

Discussion

The data demonstrate the ability of certain groups of neurons in thalamic and striopallidal nuclei to react in a detector-like fashion to a rather subtle feature of a verbal stimulus, differentiating it from others visually presented in a sequence, as being the remembered target. Both

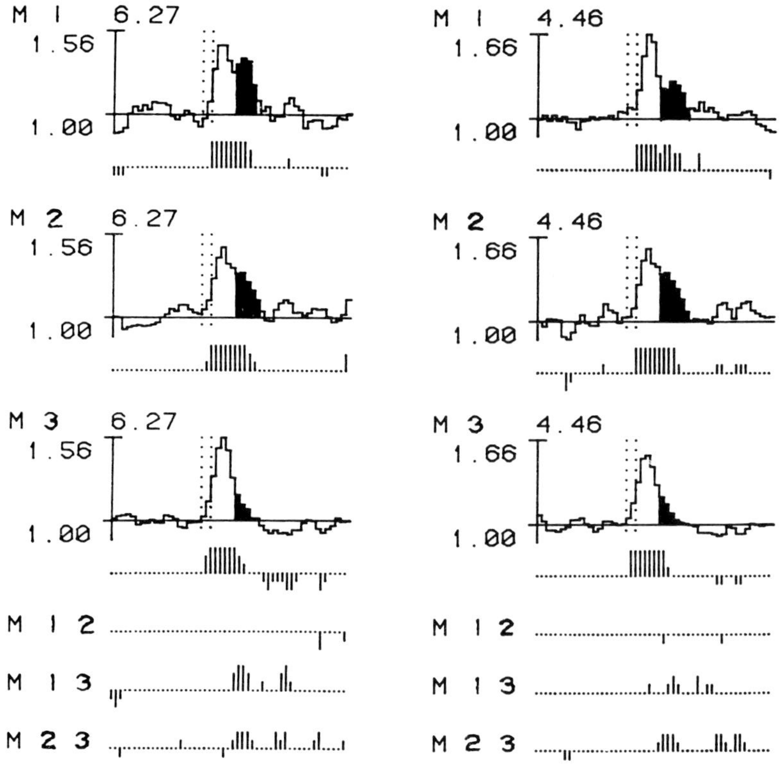

Fig. 2. Discharge rate of the neuronal population in the Vop of the thalamus (a border with Vime) of the left hemisphere during discrimination of the remembered verbal stimuli. Left and right columns of graphs contain data recorded during the two presentations to a subject of the same task with an interval of 2 days. M1 = PSTH for the trials where targets were presented; M2 = PSTH for the trials where graphically similar non-targets were presented: M3 = PSTH for the trials with dissimilar non-targets presented.

'sharply tuned' and 'broadly tuned' neurons were observed – those reacting to remembered targets only and those responding also to the graphically similar verbal stimuli. This property is not dependent upon the meaning of the stimulus, because selective responses were observed both to remembered meaningful words and to word-like meaningless quasiwords.

The results of this study make the assumption plausible that the concept of a detector neuron developed and widely used in sensory physiology may be of value in a much more general sense for understanding complicated central information processing in the brain.

Reference

1 Gogolitsin YuL, Nechaev VB: Correlates of lexical processing in the activity of neuronal populations of the human brain. Stereotact Funct Neurosurg 1990;54/55:163–167.

Yu L. Gogolitsin, MD, Institute of the Human Brain, 9, Pavlov Street,
197376 St. Petersburg (Russia)

Proceedings of the 2nd International Workshop on Microphysiological Recordings during Stereotactic Neurosurgery: Motor Thalamus, October 1–2, 1989, Nikko, Japan
Stereotact Funct Neurosurg 1993;60:152–156

Tremor and Skeletal Muscle Tone

A. Struppler

Klinikum rechts der Isar der TU München, BRD

Key Words. Stereoencephalotomy · Skeletal muscle tone · Motor control · Hypotonia · Parkinsonian tremor

Abstract. Stereotactic interventions at thalamic/subthalamic levels for parkinsonian tremor give the chance to investigate the influence of the supraspinal proprioceptive loops on the tonic component of motor tasks. Studies demonstrate not only a normalization of the late stretch reflex component and a decrease of the pre-reflex stiffness in muscles contralateral to the side of the lesion, but also a reduction of low threshold motor unit firing frequency in the elbow flexors during isometric contractions. These data indicate a shift from a more tonic to a more phasic mode of innervation, which we interpret as the cause of hypotonia.

Stereotactic interventions at thalamic/subthalamic levels for treatment of tremor provide the possibility of investigating sensory motor systems. During the intervention, experiments involving recording or stimulation in the target area provided evidence that in the target area nerve fibers are concentrated which stimulate muscle tone, presumably via the gamma system [7].

After the therapeutic lesion, two related signs of hypotonia can be observed: (1) Decreased muscular resistance to passive stretch is present in both, the relaxed and in the moderately contracting muscle. (2) Failure in rapid compensation of unexpected load perturbations is manifest in a large overshoot, particularly in the absence of visual control.

1011–6125/93/0603–0152 $ 2.75/0

Hypotonia can be caused by lesions at various levels in the somatosensory afferent system. In hypotonia of peripheral origin, i.e. sensory neuropathy, there are usually deficiencies in many somatosensory modalities and the tendon reflexes are abolished. If during the differential block, gamma axons are blocked preferentially, concomitant with other small nerve fibers, the tendon reflex disappears, due to a loss of spindle drive. In dorsal column lesions, position sense as well as vibratory sense is diminished, but the tendon reflexes remained unchanged. In hypotonia of cerebellar origin, the so-called epicritic sensitivity as well as the phasic tendon reflexes remained unchanged, but there is a combination with ataxia.

Discrete stereotactic lesions in the nucleus ventrolateralis of the thalamus (VL) and in the subthalamus can abolish resting, postural and intentional tremor. Concomitantly, rigidity is abolished and the long latency reflexe (but not the short latency) are diminished.

Reinforcement (Jendrassik' maneuver or mental drive) no longer evokes tremor or rigidity. The patient shows postural hypotonia, which is compensated by visual control, and the rebound phenomenon following sudden unloading of the muscle is pronounced. There is no deficit in maximal voluntary force or rapid movement, and no ataxia and no deficit of the so-called epicritic sensitivity can be observed. Preliminary results indicate that estimation of muscle force is disturbed.

This hypotonia of subthalamic origin seems to be for us the best model to investigate the question if there is a shift from a more tonic to a more phasic mode of innervation in hypotonia and whether this is the cause of the altered muscle tone.

Muscle tone is defined as the muscular resistence to stretch (stiffness), which is determined by (1) inherent mechanical properties of the muscle fibers, and (2) the effect of tonic innervation.

These factors are mutually related. For example, stiffness of the intrafusal fibers can modulate the threshold of the muscle spindle with subsequent effects on the stretch reflex. The influence of a preceding extension or contraction of the muscle on the sensitivity of muscle spindle primary endings and extrafusal muscle tone has recently been studied and must be taken into account when measuring muscle stiffness [2].

The experimental approach for assessment of stiffness uses torque motor devices to inflict load perturbations on contracting muscles, for example the elbow or finger flexors. Sudden load compensation corresponds to the well-known clinical rebound phenomenon.

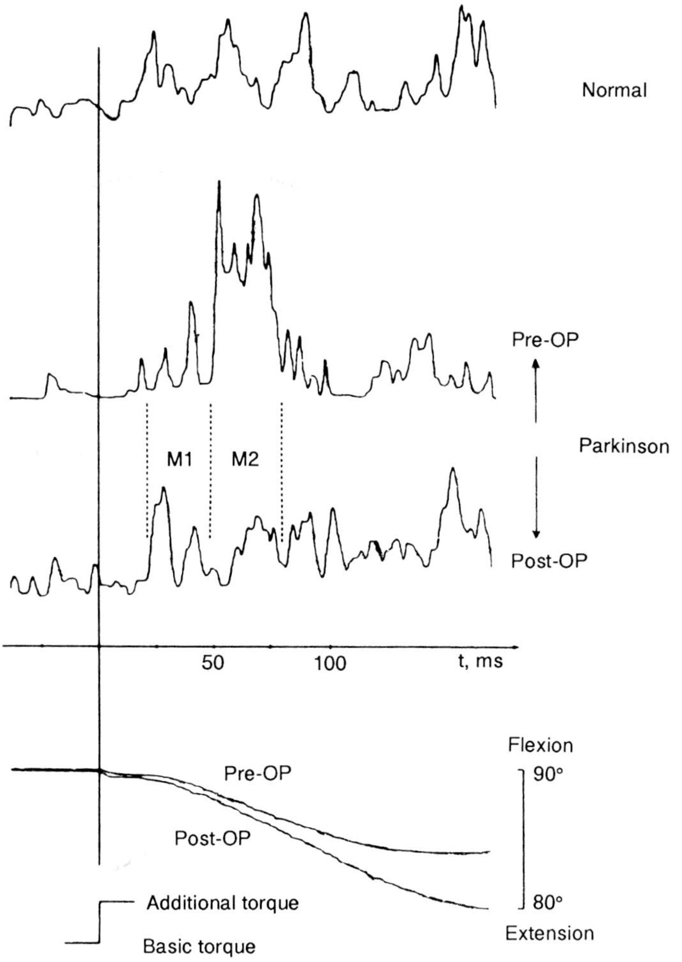

Fig. 1. M responses of the brachial muscle and displacement of the forearm following a sudden perturbation during load compensation in a patient suffering from parkinsonism before and after stereoencephalotomy. For comparison, M responses of a normal subject are depicted in the uppermost trace. Resting torque = 3.4 nm, additional torque = 3.4 nm [4].

It is known that the stretch-induced late reflex component (M2) is increased in Parkinsonian patients. In our early studies we found that it was reduced to normal in the hypotonic muscles after stereotactic treatment [3]. Additionally, we observed that torque perturbations produced a larger displacement of the limb on the hypotonic side, sometimes even prior to the onset of the phasic stretch reflex. Therefore, the question arose as to whether this type of hypotonia was primarily due to reduced 'non-reflex' muscle stiffness (fig. 1) [4].

In the case of the finger flexors, it is an advantage that the system has a relatively low inertia, which allows calculation of inertia on the basis of a linear model using viscosity and elasticity data acquired prior to the onset of the phasic stretch reflex.

All experiments were performed under the instruction 'do not intervene', in order to keep the central drive constant. Under these conditions there is no enhanced reflex excitability due to a preset and no coactivation of antagonistic muscles. Here we calculated the muscle stiffness pre- and postoperatively and observed a decrease already in the early period of the first 20 ms after the perturbation, before any reflex-electromyographic response occurred.

The early decreased muscle stiffness (pre-reflex) and the normalized late component of the stretch reflex (M2), as well as the overshoot following sudden unloading, let us speculate that the original population of motor units generating the isometric (tonic) contraction prior to the load perturbation is replaced by a different one with different intrinsic mechanical properties. In animal experiments, it could be shown that muscle stiffness depends upon the type of stimulated motor units [5].

We investigated firing frequencies of motor units activated near the recruitment level in the elbow flexor muscles. There was a significant reduction in the median firing frequency at recruitment level of around 15–20% on the operated side, compared to the opposite side or to the preoperative findings. The stability in the firing rate, however, remained unchanged.

In conclusion, stereotactic intervention for alleviation of parkinsonian tremor results not only in a normalization of the late stretch reflex component and a decrease of the pre-reflex stiffness in muscles contralateral to the side of the lesion, but also causes a reduction of low threshold motor unit firing frequency in the elbow flexors during isometric contractions.

References

1 Struppler A, Gerilovski L, Velho F, Erbel F, Altmann H: Mode of innervation following stereoencephalotomy. Contemp Clin Neurophysiol 1978;(EEG suppl 34): 493–500.

2 Jahnke MT, Proske U, Struppler A: Measurements of muscle stiffness, the electromyogram and activity in single muscle spindles of human flexor muscles following conditioning by passive stretch or contraction. Brain Res 1989;493:103–112.

3 Keidel M, Klein W, Struppler A: Stretch reflex modification by subthalatomy: A follow-up study in Parkinsonian patients. J Psychophysiol 1990;4:103–114.

4 Lehmann-Horn F, Struppler A, Klein W, Lücking CH, Burgmayer B, Deuschl G: Veränderungen der motorischen Kontrolle bei Parkinson-Patienten; in Struppler A (ed): Elektrophysiologische Diagnostik in der Neurologie. Thieme, Stuttgart, 1982, pp 236–237.

5 Petit J, Filippi GM, Emonet-Denand F, Hunt CC, Laporte Y: Changes in muscle stiffness produced by motor units of different types in peroneus longus muscle of cat. J Neurophysiol 1990;63:190–197.

A. Struppler, MD, Klinikum rechts der Isar der TU München,
Ismaninger Strasse 22, D-W-8000 München 80 (FRG)

Announcements

International Workshop on Microphysiological Recording

The 'Third International Workshop on Microphysiological Recording during Stereotactic Neurosurgery: Microelectrode Recording in Man' has been scheduled for October 10, 1993 at the Stouffer's El Presidente Hotel in Mexico City, immediately prior to the XIth Meeting of the World Society for Stereotactic and Functional Neurosurgery in Ixtapa, Mexico.

For additional information, please contact: Ronald R. Tasker, MD, MA, FRCS (C), The Toronto Hospital, Toronto Western Division, Suite 2–431, McLaughlin Pavilion, 399 Rathurst Street, Toronto, Ontario M5T 2S8 (Canada).

Phone: 416–369–5571. FAX: 416–369–5298.

World Society for Stereotactic and Functional Neurosurgery

The XIth Meeting of the World Society for Stereotactic and Functional Neurosurgery will be held at the Ixtapa Westin Hotel in Ixtapa, Mexico, October 11–15, 1993, which is immediately before the October 10, 1993 meeting of the World Federation of Neurosurgical Societies in Acapulco, Mexico.

For additional information, please contact: Philip L. Gildenberg, MD, PhD, 6560 Fannin – Suite 1530, Houston, TX 77030 (USA).

Phone: 713–790–0795. FAX: 713–669–0388.